Forms of Psychological Inquiry

Critical Assessments of Contemporary Psychology
A Series of Columbia University Press
Daniel N. Robinson, Series Editor

Forms of Psychological Inquiry

Joseph M. Notterman

Columbia University Press   New York   1985

Library of Congress Cataloging in Publication Data

Notterman, Joseph M.

Forms of psychological inquiry.
(Critical Assessments of Contemporary Psychology)
Bibliography: p.
Includes index.
1. Psychology—Methodology.   I. Title   II. Series
BF38.5.N67 1985   150'.1   84-23035
ISBN 0-231-05988-4

Columbia University Press
New York   Guildford, Surrey
Copyright © 1985 Columbia University Press
All rights reserved

Printed in the United States of America

Clothbound editions of Columbia University Press books
are Smyth-sewn and printed on permanent and durable
acid-free paper.

For my granddaughter, Arielle Leah Notterman,
on her first birthday.

Contents

Acknowledgments

I appreciate the helpful suggestions made by the several under-graduate and graduate students who read portions of this book as it was being written. Among them are Scott Janney, Debbie Schade, Diane Schiano, and Arthur Whaley. Jeanette Koffler typed the first draft from tapes, and Arlene Kronewitter turned the subsequent drafts into final copy. Michael Ticktin assisted with identification of biblical sources; Marilyn Ticktin, with proofreading. Dr. Benjamin B. Wolman offered constructive comments on the manuscript as a whole, particularly with regard to the chapters on psychoanalysis. It was my good fortune to have David Diefendorf as manuscript editor; the finished work owes much to his competence. Professor Daniel N. Robinson, the series editor, was always available; he guided without directing.

As in all things, my family was quietly supportive.

Preface

The foremost aim of this book is to assist the student of psychology in gaining a perspective on the field. By "perspective" I mean the following: First, the recognition that many of the problems we consider to be new in psychology are really quite old—some even primeval in origin. Second, the realization that even though these problems exist, our understanding of them, and of their relation to each other, keeps changing and is gradually but steadily increasing. By maintaining our perspective, we make neither a fetish of the past, nor a fad of the present.

In order to achieve this aim, the chapters are conceived and the references selected so as to capture psychology's rich diversity. Topics are considered that range from the basic to the applied, from the established to the speculative, from the experimental to the clinical.

The book departs from the conventional history and systems text in several ways: (1) It avoids as much as possible a linear account of historical events in psychology. My concern is not with "history" or "schools" per se, but with integrating and consolidating the materials to which we have been exposed in various areas of psychology. (2) It endeavors to cultivate a respect for *all* forms of psychological inquiry, because each viewpoint has its own merits. Our task is to appreciate the *reasons* behind the various viewpoints. (3) Of the *how* (methodology) and *what* (facts) of each form of psychological inquiry, only enough is given to afford a basis for asking the *why* (reasons) for its existence. In each chapter, I have screened what is ordinarily contained in a history and systems book, and drawn attention to major issues that seem to me to have been neglected. In this sense, the chapters are really essays. (4) The book quotes liberally from original works and from reference sources. In part, this was done to be as precise as possible. In addition, this tactic was employed because it cannot be taken for granted that the original works or reference sources are readily available to the student. (5) An emphasis is given to problems of psychotherapy, and to what I perceive as a growing eclecticism in approach to treatment. Special concern for this topic seemed warranted, given the prevalence of mental disorders in the United States, and the number of students entering into one or another of the therapeutic fields.

Depending upon the nature of the course for which this book is assigned, the book may be used as a text. Alternatively, it may be used either with additional reading material selected by the instructor, or in conjunction with a standard history and systems text.

Forms of Psychological Inquiry evolved over several years during which I taught a course bearing the same title at Princeton University. It was an enjoyable challenge. I hope the lessons I learned are reflected in these pages.

Forms of Psychological Inquiry

1 Cosmology, Spirits, and Animism: Origins and Continuing Influence

The first objective of this chapter is to conjecture as carefully as possible about primitive man's ideas of himself, of others, and of the environment. The second objective is to suggest how some of these archaic views influence modern man's conceptions of behavior. In working toward these objectives, we shall depend upon scraps of evidence and plain guesswork. These stem from diverse disciplines such as etymology, anthropology, archeology, learning theory, and psychoanalysis. If we are cautious in our interpretations, the effort should be intellectually satisfying, even though we can never know for certain that our surmises have been correct. Our higher purpose is to cultivate a feeling of empathy with past generations of mankind, and a sense of awe at their accomplishments.

Derivation of "Psychology"

The prefix to the word psychology derives from the ancient Greek "psyche" which meant breath, spirit, soul, or mind. Breath, spirit, soul, mind—what is the relation among them? The gist of this chapter is that well before the Greeks, the necessary relation of breath to primeval man's *own* capacity for action gave

rise over eons to the idea of spirit. Over the course of further mil-
lenia, two refinements occurred: the idea of spirit led to the concept of soul in religion, and of mind in philosophy and psychology. As we shall see, elements of primeval man's conceptions of
himself, and of the universe about him, have persisted down to
the present through language, culture, and religion.

Homo Sapiens and His Rudimentary Cosmology

What do we know of the earliest man? Actually, very
little. *Homo sapiens* evolved in Europe or Central Asia (possibly
concurrently in both places) about 250,000 years ago.[1] In terms
relative to that of *geological* time, man is of recent existence. It has
been observed that:

if the whole of earth's history were "compressed into a single year," the
scale of our physical evolution to the present would be something like
this: the first eight months would be completely without life; the following two months would be devoted to the most primitive of creatures;
mammals would not appear before the second week of December; man,
as we know him, would strut onto the stage at approximately 11:45 p.m.
on December 31. The age of written history would occupy little more
than the last sixty seconds on the clock.[2]

From skull fragments found at various sites, it appears that early *Homo sapiens'* brain capacity was similar to ours.
Remnants of stone and flint artifacts indicate that he crafted tools.
The locations of these sites, as well as the particular quantities
of artifacts found at them, suggest that he hunted in small (probably single-family) bands, the so-called "primeval horde."
His view of the world has been described as "cosmological," but without at all connoting the intellectualized, mystical concept of "ordered whole" or "harmonious universe," a
meaning given to the term "cosmos" by the Indo-Aryan and Greek
thinkers.[3] Rather, primeval man's outlook was cosmological only
in the sense that he did not draw a cognitive distinction between

nonbiological and biological aspects of the world. The earth and the air were thought to be just as alive as he. Perhaps this was so because the quality of being "alive" was equated to the capacity for action. Thus, spontaneous changes in terrestrial stability, as in earthquakes, or in the intensity or direction of air, as in windstorms, imparted the quality of what *we* call "life" to the earth and to the air. The presence of action, regardless of its cause, blurred the distinction between nonbiological and biological entities and processes. A cat stalking a wind-blown object, the way it would a mouse, illustrates the point.

Purpose-behind-action

We may further conjecture that primeval man assumed that there was purpose-behind-action. Since *he* usually did not initiate action (be it hunting, feeding, playing, grooming, or mating) unless he had some definite purpose, he attributed intent to any action he observed, regardless of the entity involved. So, for example, the sun was "alive" because it appeared to move itself in an orbit across the sky. The purpose of the sun's action "must be" to bring day and night, and the seasons. The tendency to infer purpose from action—whether or not logically—is still very much with us today, as subsequent chapters demonstrate.

Reification of Breathing Process into Spirit

Our distant forebear must have noticed that there was only one circumstance in which the initiation of action ceased *permanently*, and that was when breathing also ceased. This was true of the animals he killed while hunting, as well as of his fellow primates who died an accidental or natural death. Further, the permanent cessation of the breathing process could be explained by the possibility that some *thing* had departed from the body.

Early man reified (i.e., made a thing out of) the breath which left the body at death, and called it "spirit."

Etymological considerations support this conjecture, since the word spirit derives from the archaic Latin "spirare," meaning "to breathe." The modern Hebrew word for soul, "neshama," derives from the pre-Biblical Hebrew, "neshima," meaning "breath."[4]

Of course, primeval man did not possess language as we know it. In using etymological sources to inquire about the origins of "spirit," we are not only leaping tens of thousands of years before early man's time, but we are assuming that the roots of words can reflect what were initially nonverbal, protocognitive preoccupations with the universe.[5]

Dreams and Wandering Spirit

Abetting the idea of spirit was the observation that action could cease in man and animals for substantial periods of time, *without* an accompanying cessation of breathing. An obvious instance was that of sleep. And during sleep, man experienced the visual, auditory, kinesthetic, and other imagery of dreaming. He would wander far and wide in space, or go back and forth in time, and yet awake to find his body in the same spot as when he first fell asleep. The imagery of dreaming may have been indistinguishable from the imagery of remembering, and probably appeared just as real to him. Such dream-experiences facilitated a conceptualization of spirit as a thing able to leave the body not only permanently, but temporarily as well.

What were the characteristics attributed to this "thing"? Simply enough, spirit was endowed with those behavioral properties which man knew best; namely, his own. The first "inner man" or psychological homunculus was born. Homunculus is a term popularized in modern times by B. F. Skinner. He uses this word to point to cases where both laymen and scientists reify the processes underlying natural phenomena, and thereby claim that they have provided an explanation.

Relations among Spirits, Homunculi, and Animism

Spirit had attained virtual autonomy. Once it was conceived as an inner person, it possessed the ability to behave in its own right. Spirit had its own identity, one separate from its possessor. Primeval man was now in a position to leap forward in his conception of the universe. He could explain how the sun and the earth had purpose to their actions, even though they were not obvious breathing-entities. They were inhabited by spirits! Of even greater fundamental importance: once the idea of an autonomous spirit took hold, the concept was generalized to all entities and processes, whether or not they were characterized by the capacity for spontaneous change. There was a spirit in a peaceful mountain, just as there was in an erupting volcano. Spirits occupied every object and accounted for every phenomenon.

Although man served as the prototype, the behavioral characteristics of a particular spirit were eventually modified so as to resemble those of its unique possessor. For example, the spirit which inhabited the earth became known as "mother nature," since it normally provided "maternal" nourishment in the form of wild berries, fruits, and grains.

The spirit view of the world is called *animism*, the belief that all natural objects and phenomena possess spirits. (Granted all the foregoing conjectures, it should come as no surprise that "animism" descends from the ancient Latin "anim(a)," meaning "air, the breath of life, spirit. . . .") As noted earlier, animism is a rudimentary form of cosmology. Cosmology is the conception of the world as an orderly system, without regard to whether the parts or processes comprising the system are organic or inorganic. If all entities and functions possess spirits, then the mysteries of existence and of the world are thereby solved, and by means of an orderly, unifying principle.

Neanderthal Man and Deification

Neanderthal man—the colloquially named "cave-man"—came on the scene about 75,000 years ago. He hunted in multifamilial bands. Not only did he believe in spirits, but the awesome idea of an afterlife had emerged. When a spirit left him permanently, it had to go *somewhere*. Sample evidence is provided by the results of archeological excavations in France during the twentieth century:

A boy about fifteen or sixteen years old had been buried in a cave. He had been lowered into a trench, placed on his right side with knees slightly drawn and head resting on his forearm in a sleeping position. A pile of flints lay under his head to form a sort of stone pillow, and near his hand was a beautiful worked stone ax. Around the remains were wild-cattle bones, many of them charred, the remnants of roasted meat which may have been provided to serve as sustenance in the world of the dead.[6]

Reification, in the form of animism, was eventually followed by the elevation of major spirits to the level of deities. For example, Ra became the Egyptian spirit-god of the sun; and possibly because of the importance to terrestrial life of the sun's light and heat, he also became the principal god of ancient Egypt. For the Greeks, "mother nature" was formalized as Demeter, the goddess of the fruitful earth, and subsequently, of fruitful marriage. The concept of spirit was not abandoned; gods and goddesses were assigned control over them. Early religions had roles for both.

In the ancient East, spirit evolved mainly into what we mean today by "soul," and partly into "mind." In the ancient West, the balance was the other way around; spirit became primarily "mind," partially "soul." And in that portion of the world lying in between, there eventually was a synthesis of the concepts of spirit, soul, mind, and deity—the idea of a single Supreme Being.

Continuing Influence of Animism

It would be a mistake to assume that animism is no longer both prevalent and influential, despite the evolution of monotheistic religion. For example, animism (together with the ancient breathing ritual of yoga) is at the core of Hinduism, the dominant religion of modern India. In terms of world membership, the adherents of the Hindu religion vie with those of the Muslim religion for second place after Christianity. Thus one of today's most important faiths is a religion of reification and of breathing-regulated, meditative practices, with a firm belief in spirits.[7]

We Westerners, too, have been influenced by reification and animism. We sing "Old Man River." We say, "My parking-lot sticker has expired." We complain, "The computer has gone crazy." We advertise, "The spirit of Marlboro in a low tar cigarette" (depicted as a cowboy on a horse). And we give individuality to hurricanes by assigning names to them.

Cro-Magnon's Cave Paintings and the First Totem

By the time of the Cro-Magnon (about 35,000 years ago) people approaching ourselves had evolved. Our knowledge of them is based largely upon excavations in France and Spain, although it is thought that they came there from the eastern (or opposite) side of the Mediterranean. They lived in tribes consisting of several multifamilial bands. They were the first to develop art, which took the form of lasting paintings on cave walls. These paintings depict humans, animals, and an unusual type of symbol known as a "totem."

Cro-Magnon went through the labor of searching out natural dyes which he could then use in the attempt to create *permanent* pictures. Why? Possibly the paintings were yet another manifestation of reification and deification. The spirits and demigods in this case were the visual images which comprise so much of the processes that we call "memory" and "fantasy." We recollect the face of a friend, or of our favorite childhood dog, in our "mind's eye." Similarly, Cro-Magnon recalled the tribal leaders, the fellow-hunters, and the animals that sustained him in the days or years past. We take these images for granted; Cro-Magnon probably marveled at them.

He reified the fleeting images by painting them on the walls of certain of his caves. Thereby, they were "stored," and became available upon need. These caves are almost inaccessible. Their remoteness suggests that they were considered to be holy ground. The paintings themselves are thought to have been revered.[8] A. Marshack has noted the following by way of describing a museum exhibition entitled "Ice Age Art: 35,000–10,000 B.C."

These and other animal images were not simply illustrations. They had become symbols, they stood for processes in nature and they had probably become mythologized. Quite often they played a role in ritual, religion and story. Animal images could apparently be used in ceremonies of many kinds, perhaps in a curing ceremony, or to mark an important life event such as birth or even death, or to honor the coming of spring.[9]

The artistic efforts of the Cro-Magnon peoples were not limited to the cave-paintings found in France and Spain, where the ecology facilitated this particular mode of creative endeavor.

Ice Age artists developed almost every technique of artistic production possible for a Stone Age hunter and achieved mastery in each of these techniques. These included carving in the round and bas-relief of stone, bone, ivory, and clay, and engraving or line drawing in the same materials. . . . Even the polishing of stone and the firing of clay were mastered in some areas. . . . A prehistoric kiln for firing clay statues of animals and females . . . found in . . . Czechoslovakia, confirms the development of a regional technology for art, as advanced as any developed for painting in the French and Spanish caves.[10]

Nor was music neglected. "Two flutes, each with six holes—four above and two below—found in France and Russia document the presence of true, tonal music."[11] Accordingly, it is tempting to conjecture that Cro-Magnon man, just as modern man, possessed an artistic impulse independently of any ritualistic motivation.

Eventually, the *totem* was created. It was a symbol designed to represent the collective spirit of a given tribe. The totem claimed allegiance and respect, much as the flag of a nation, or the emblem of a religion does today.

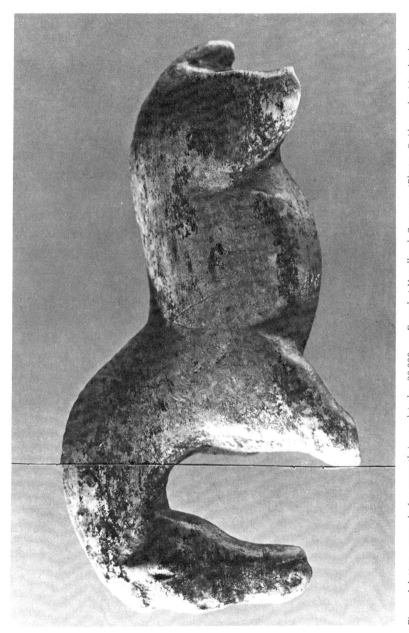

Figure 1.1 Horse carved of mammoth ivory, dated c. 30,000 B.C. Found at Vogelherd, Germany. (Photo: © Alexander Marshack)

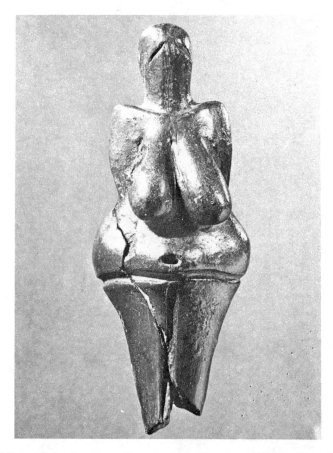

Figure 1.2 Female figurine ("Venus") made of fired clay, dated 27,000 B.C. Found at Dolni Vestonici, Czechoslavakia. (Photo: © Alexander Marshack)

Freud's *Totem and Taboo*, and Hate-honor Ambivalence

In *Totem and taboo*, Freud made use of his own clinical observations and psychoanalytic assumptions, together with anthropological interpretations, to derive the following understanding of the totem's utility.[12]

Beginning with the Neanderthal period, each horde was dominated by a mature, male ruler. He maintained his status by either castrating or killing any younger males who challenged his sexual or other prerogatives. As generations went by, the sons developed ways to cope with the paternal threat. They learned to leave the horde upon reaching puberty, and to establish their own familial groups. But before doing so, the sons banded together and killed and ate the father! By our standards, such cannibalistic patricide is almost unbelievable. Freud reminds us, however, that we are considering a period in the human being's evolution when he was as much a beast as he was a human. Freud also argued that the act of eating the father was not entirely hostile in nature. He held that the behavior was also based upon the processes of identification and incorporation, and thus was a way of "honoring" the paternal figure through having the father become part of the son.

The same cycle was repeated with each newly formed horde. Eventually, social rules (or taboos) were developed to resolve the hate-honor ambivalence which the sons felt toward the father. Instead of incorporating the father, a totem feast was held. Freud asserted that through displacement, a living animal was substituted for the father's flesh and spirit, then killed and eaten. Eventually, the cathartic acting-out of ambivalence toward the father went beyond that of the totem feast. The acting-out included the periodic destruction of carved, sculpted, or painted idols of tribal gods. The fallen idol was then replaced with another, whose greater power and love might bring greater fortune to the tribe. But hate-honor ambivalence toward the parental figure remained as the basis for such behavior.

Freud extended his psychoanalytic conjectures to include the evolution of religion in general, and of Christianity in particular. He wrote:

The religion of the son succeeds the religion of the father. As a sign of this substitution the old totem feast is revived again in the form of communion in which the band of brothers now eats the flesh and blood of the son and no longer that of the father, the sons thereby identifying themselves with him and becoming holy themselves. Thus through the ages we see the identity of the totem feast with the animal sacrifice, the theanthropic human sacrifice, and the Christian eucharist, and in all these solemn occasions we recognize the after-effects of that crime which so oppressed men but of which they must have been so proud. At bottom, however, the Christian communion is a new setting aside of the father, a repetition of the crime that must be expiated. We see how well justified is Frazer's dictum that "the Christian communion has absorbed within itself a sacrament which is doubtless far older than Christianity." [13]

Whether or not Freud's claim is warranted, we should bear in mind that religious conviction and psychological understanding are not at all mutually exclusive. [14]

For purposes of meeting the objectives of this chapter, we have delved sufficiently into cosmology, spirits, and animism. We recognize that there is not a clear-cut progression from breath to spirit, soul, or mind. Many variables affected the selection of the particular processes that were reified, and the sequences with which such reification, and sometimes deification, occurred. However, the fact that there was *any* relation at all, regardless of whether it was a progression, needs to be explored. For as already indicated, these ideas have had an important influence—a lasting influence—upon the character of forms of psychological inquiry yet to be examined.

2 Structuralism: Ancient and Modern Mind-Body Dualisms

This chapter's overall objective is to provide a perspective on structuralism, through considering this school in the context of its having served as a transition between ancient and modern mind-body dualisms. To achieve this aim, the chapter begins by continuing with our examination of man's evolution, especially in regard to his psychological development. It then goes on to describe the beginning of scientific method. Finally, the chapter presents and evaluates the chief contributions made by structuralism's originators and elaborators, and by recent students of consciousness.

The Continuing Evolution of Man:
Ecological, Social, and Economic Factors

With the passage of generations, ecological factors became of increasing importance to man's psychological development. The type of home he found or built, the mores he established, the reinforcement contingencies he encountered—even the quality of his consciousness—all these were affected by the particular environmental configuration within which he and his tribespeople interacted. Thus, one settlement became quite different from another—different, yet affected by the same parameters. For example, the rich soil of the Nile delta invited agricultural pursuits. The river itself enabled ready transportation between villages, thereby permitting distribution of produce. The exchange of produce for other commodities led to the development of trading centers and commercialization. The coming together of otherwise isolated people became an occasion for festivities and cultural enrichment. The more important of these foci of civilization became capitals, often rivaling each other for the prestige and profit that attended such status.

Variations of this particular prototype existed in the "fertile crescent" formed by the Tigris and Euphrates, in the valley of the Indus, and in the alluvial surrounds of the Ganges. Relative to the modes of transportation then available, vast distances separated these areas. But, as we shall see later, routes existed whereby contact (either friendly or hostile) could have been made among them.

Other cultural prototypes were determined by the presence of lakes and inland seas, by forests and mountains, and by bordering seas and oceans. For instance, the Aegean Sea separated a European outpost from an Asian one. Homer's epics describe the resulting clash that took place about 3,200 years ago. The geographical and cultural-political parameters which affected the onset and course of the Trojan War have been crisply summarized by G. Highet as follows:

Geographically, the world of the poems is fairly narrow. It is wider than the world we see through the early books of the Old Testament, but still it is limited: mainland Greece; the western coast of Asia Minor; Crete and Cyprus; Phoenicia; Egypt; the Greek islands; and beyond these a realm where reality merges into fantasy . . . politically, it is not a society of countries with national boundaries as we know them, but of cities and tribes. There are no "Greeks." There is a strong tribe which inhabits southern Greece and which draws allies from elsewhere. It is called the Achaeans . . . it is besieging Troy.

Troy is a single city in northwestern Asia Minor near the Dardanelles. It is ancient and powerful and rich . . . its king Priam is an Oriental sultan with a harem, and he has brought in allies from elsewhere in Asia.[1]

Of course, we all know how the Trojan War purportedly came to an end. It was through the sly use of an animal totem.

What is "Real"?

The central point of the foregoing account of differing sites of civilization is that each such zone developed its own conceptualization of reality. Even more so than today, the individual who traveled from one environmental domain to another must have experienced a severe challenge to his basic assumptions of what is *real*, of what is universally lasting. The gods and goddesses of one culture were different from those of another. Behaviors that were correct in Greece were barbaric in Egypt (and vice-versa) even though only a few hundred miles separated the two civilizations.

Plato's Exodus

And so it might have been with Plato, when a change in political regime (about 400 B.C.) compelled him to leave Athens at age 28. In brief, his exile came about as follows: By Plato's time, Athens had grown to be a metropolis of some 400,000 persons, of whom 250,000 were slaves, and 150,000 were free men. The 30-year war with Sparta had just been lost. In the ensuing unrest, two major political parties vied for power. One favored a populist type of democracy, and held sway; the other favored an oligarchy ruled by an intellectual aristocracy. The latter party incited a revolution, which was unsuccessful. Socrates was the intellectual leader of this group; he was imprisoned and put to trial. Convicted, he was sentenced to drink poison. Friends arranged for a convenient escape, but Socrates refused. He was only 70 and could look forward to the fruits of ripening years, but he accepted his fate.

Plato had been among those of Socrates' students who had attempted to save the master's life. His own was now in danger. And so he left Athens. Where did he go? One speculation is particularly interesting.

He seems to have gone first to Egypt; and was somewhat shocked to hear from the priestly class which ruled that land, that Greece was an infant-state, without stabilizing traditions or profound culture, not yet therefore to be taken seriously by these sphinxly pundits of the Nile. . . . And then off he sailed to Sicily, and to Italy; there he joined for a time the school or sect which the great Pythagoras had founded. . . . Twelve years he wandered, imbibing wisdom from every source, sitting at every shrine, tasting every creed. Some would have it that he went to Judea and was moulded for a while by the tradition of the almost socialistic prophets; and even that he found his way to the banks of the Ganges, and learned the mystic meditations of the Hindus. We do not know.[2]

Transportation Links Between Ancient West and East

Was it indeed feasible for Plato to have traveled as widely as has been speculated? At issue is not so much whether Plato himself or any one individual made the *entire* trip to the Far East, as it is to recognize that transportation links between the ancient East and West existed to a far greater extent than we ordinarily realize. Further, we must recognize that the consequences of early intercultural communication continue to affect our present psychological views of human behavior, through the folklore, literature, religions, and philosophies passed down to us.

Using Athens as a point of departure, there are three major water-caravan routes whereby the actual or an invented Plato could have made his way to India. There are shown by the dashed lines on the map. The routes numbered "1" and "2" are extensions of water routes used for trading purposes by the Cretans as far back as 1,450 B.C. Cretan artwork and other relics have been found in Egypt, and vice versa. Peoples of the eastern Mediterranean also sailed to Troy and to the Island of Cyprus; and past

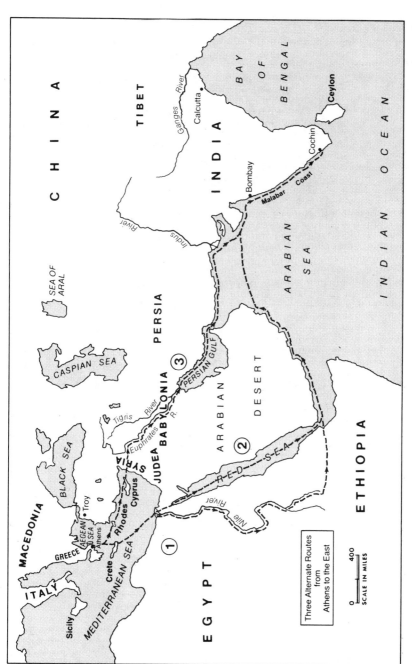

Figure 2.1 Three geographical lines of communication between ancient West and East.

Cyprus to Phoenicia (approximately the coast of Judea). Camel and donkey caravans were used to bridge the land masses across Ethiopia, as well as those between the Mediterranean Sea and the Red Sea. By hugging the southern coast of Arabia, and by venturing across the Persian Gulf or the Arabian Sea, landfall could be made near the Indus River. Route "3" shows how, by means of island-hopping, contact could be made with Judea; and how caravan routes led to the Euphrates River, and then beyond to the Persian Gulf and to the coasts of Persia and India.

Additional evidence that it was possible for Plato to have traveled as far as India is contained in the following journalist's dispatch sent to the *New York Times* from Cochin, a town on the Malabar Coast of southwest India.

"The first Jews in India are believed to have arrived on the Malabar Coast in this state of Kerala on King Solomon's merchant fleet in 973 B.C." (Recall that King Solomon traded with Ethiopia via the Red Sea. His marriage to the Queen of Sheba may have been inspired by economics and politics as much as by romance!) "Some scholars say that the Jews . . . settled about 25 miles north of Cochin, after the conquest of Judea by Babylon in 586 B.C."[3] The Bible itself implies that Hebrews had direct or indirect trade relations with India. In the Song of Songs (1:13), the woman narrator says: "While the king was reclining on his board, my nard sent forth its fragrance." Nard is "an aromatic Himalayan plant, believed to be the spikenard, . . . the source of an ointment used by the ancients."[4] The Himalayan Mountains, of course, separate Tibet from India.

Plato left Athens about 400 B.C. If the Israelites could have made their way to India at least two and possibly six centuries before, not only could he, should he have been so disposed, but so could others of whom much less is known.

Platonic Idealism and Mind-matter Dualism

By the time of Plato's studies with Socrates, the essentials of most modern civilized thought had been explored, debated, accepted, rejected, and reconsidered. However, Plato's idealism seems to have been uniquely his own creation. Idealism asserts the existence of "universals" or "forms" which inhere in themselves, and are independent of the biases or perceptions of any particular individual. For instance, the *idea* of "beauty" is an abstraction which transcends particularity. However, what is specifically perceived as being beautiful will vary from person to person, from time to time, and from culture to culture. Similarly, the idea of "circularity" is mathematically pure, even though no perfect circle can ever be drawn regardless of the means employed.

Ideas or forms or universals endure forever. Accordingly, they constitute reality. The objects of our material world eventually all decay. Therefore, if knowledge is to be based upon reality, it must be based upon ideas, and not upon unique, physical representations of them.

Ideas were also basic to Plato's distinction between consciousness and mind. Consciousness consists merely of amorphous or unstructured stimulation from the senses. The mind is comprised of the *coherence* or structure brought to consciousness through ideas. Ideas are made available through thinking and then utilized by reasoning. Without ideas, and the life-continuing influence of ideas, there could be no mind.

Edna Heidbreder pulled together, in elegantly concise fashion, Platonic idealism and mind-matter dualism:

Plato formulated . . . the clear-cut distinction between mind and matter that has figured prominently in psychology down to the present time. . . . Plato . . . gave himself over as completely as possible to the life of reason . . . he was deeply impressed by the difference between *ideas*, which are revealed by reason, and *things*, which are revealed by the senses; and placing ideas in a world by themselves, he regarded them as far more real than the world known to the senses.[5]

Descartes's "Cognitive Soul" and Mind-body Interactionism

Descartes restored some balance. Whereas Platonic mind-body dualism was completely philosophic and exempted

science, Cartesian mind-body dualism provided the foundation for
a physiological psychology.

For Descartes, consciousness was an awareness of
thought or mind. Thought *itself* was reality. It was the only aspect
of life whose existence could not be doubted (hence, "I think,
therefore I am.") Thought included the inevitable emergence of
certain ideas, such as God, self, and mathematical relations. Descartes was an intensely religious man, a devout French Catholic.
For him, as well as for many other philosophers and scientists
throughout history, the idea of God was beyond, and did not even
require, logical proof. The idea was immanent; for Descartes, it
was a dominant idea latent in all human beings. In short, Descartes's view of "mind" is almost as if the mind were a thinking
or cognitive *soul*, one which established personal identity through
thought.

In order for the cognitive soul to rule the body, it had
to have means whereby material events of the outside world were
translated into actions dictated by the soul's will or volition. Descartes's mechanical-hydraulic theory of input-output reflex action
served as the necessary model. It was a model that satisfied his
scientific obligations as a "modest materialist," his philosophical
position, as well as his religious beliefs.[6] His notion of the sensory-motor arc served for both humans and animals. But animals
were like automata or robots, or machines. They had no purpose
or volition or will, since they had no souls, a position strictly in
accord with Descartes's religious convictions.

As we shall see, Plato's and Descartes's rationalist views
of consciousness and mind influenced the scientific work of the
structuralist school in psychology. Structuralism could not have
begun to run its course, however, in the absence of Kant's, Comte's,
and Helmoltz's contributions. (Tables 2.1 and 2.2 are provided to
assist in keeping terminology and ideas straight while increasing
contact is made with structuralism.)

Table 2.1 Some basic philosophical terms in juxtaposition. (Derived from a variety of sources)

ON ULTIMATES AND SCIENTIFIC METHODOLOGY

Theology & Metaphysics: Theology—The field of study and analysis which treats of God and His relation to the universe. Metaphysics—the philosophical inquiry into ultimates, or fundamental truth, or reality.

Positivism: A philosophical system advanced by Auguste Comte, concerned with explicitly stated facts and phenomena, and excluding speculation upon ultimate causes or origins; the restriction of inquiry to problems open to scientific methods.

ON REALITY

Idealism: The doctrine that ideas and thought constitute the fundamental reality.

Materialism: The doctrine that matter is the only reality.

ON KNOWLEDGE

Rationalism: The doctrine that reason alone is the major source of knowledge and is independent of experience. ("Cognizance," or thought, in consciousness.)

Empiricism: The doctrine that all knowledge is derived from experience. ("Awareness," or sensation and feeling, in consciousness.)

Beginnings of Scientific Method: Kant, Comte, and Helmholtz

In his *Critique of Pure Reason,* the German philosopher Immanuel Kant held that consciousness is determined jointly by sensations and by certain innate characteristics of mind. His view of ideas as innate attributes was more sophisticated than either Plato's or Descartes's. They consisted of an intuition of space and time, a tendency to seek causality or organization among events, and a capacity to apperceive. Apperception is the ability to develop a new perception by assimilating current knowledge and experience with previous knowledge and experience. In a word, apperception is the ability to modify one's previous perceptions.

As to the study of consciousness itself, Kant was pessimistic. He believed that it was impossible to know pure consciousness, since to do so, the mind is involved, and imposes itself upon the inquiry. How telling is this criticism of introspection

Table 2.2 Major contributors to the evolution and decline of structuralism and their particular philosophical emphases.

Each contributor's position is indicated by "X" if strongly protagonist, or by "Some," if moderately so. Those whose names are underlined are Structuralists proper.

	Ultimates & Sci. Method		Reality		Knowledge		Key Contribution
	Theology & Metaphysics	Positivism	Idealism	Materialism	Rationalism	Empiricism	
Plato (427–347 B.C.)	X	—	X	—	X	—	Mind-Matter Dualism
Descartes (1596–1650)	X	—	X	Some	X	Some	Interactionism; "cognitive" soul
Kant (1724–1804)	Some	—	X	Some	Some	Some	Innate ideas of causality; apperception
Comte (1798–1857)	—	X	—	X	—	X	Philosophical founder of Positivism
Weber (1795–1878)	—	X	—	X	—	X	$\Delta S/S = $ constant $=$ jnd of sensation
Fechner (1801–1887)	X	X	—	X	—	X	sensation $= k \log S + c$; cosmologist
Helmholtz (1821–1894)	—	X	—	X	—	X	Doctrine: "mind" is reducible to materialistic events
Wundt (1832–1920)	—	X	—	X	—	X	Parallelism: first formal psych. lab, Leipsig
Kulpe (1862–1915)	—	X	Some	Some	Some	Some	Imageless thought; unconscious reasoning; Wurzburg School
Titchener (1867–1927)	—	X	Some	Some	Some	Some	Core-Context Theory of Meaning; abandonment of traditional Structuralism

as a means whereby consciousness may be studied? It depends upon whether the inquiry is anchored to some set of operations which specify and manipulate consciousness *independently* of consciousness itself. The persons who made this point were Comte and Helmholtz.

Auguste Comte's *Law of Three Stages* describes the way explanations of natural and social phenomena have progressed during the course of human development. The French founder of positivism calls these natural and social phenomena "subjects."

At first the subject was conceived in the *theological* fashion, and all problems were explained by the will of some deity . . . as when the stars were gods, or the chariots of gods; later, the same subject reached the *metaphysical* stage, and was explained by metaphysical abstractions—as when the stars moved in perfect circles because circles were the most perfect figure; finally the subject was reduced to *positive* science by precise observation, hypothesis, and experiment, and its phenomena were explained through the regularities of natural cause and effect.[7]

Comte initiated positivist thinking to philosophy and to science.

Hermann von Helmholtz, in the doctrine which bears his name, carried to the limit the application of positivism to psychology. In straightforward materialist fashion, he held that sensation and mind itself *must* be reduced to physiological, physical, or chemical events. A strict interpretation of the Helmholtz Doctrine implies that psychology, whether considered as either a behavioristic or a cognitive discipline (to take two extreme viewpoints), is concerned merely with epiphenomena. We shall see, when we examine Russian psychology, that the Helmholtz Doctrine is equivalent to what Marx and Lenin later called "one-way dialectical materialism."

Definitions of Stimulus, Sensation, and Perception

One additional step must be taken before we can turn our attention to the structuralists proper, and that is to define the terms "stimulus," "sensation," and "perception." A cautionary word is essential, if we are not to fall victim to fruitless dispute. As Woodworth remarks in opening the discussion of "Sensation and Perception" in his classic text, *Experimental Psychology*, "If we should attempt to begin this study with an adequate definition of these terms, we should find ourselves in the midst of a debate that has gone on for many generations of psychologists and philosophers."[8] So let us agree to abide by the following definitions, although others may be equally valid. These are offered because they are fairly compatible with the ones used by the structuralists.

Stimulus: A physical or chemical agent acting through an appropriate receiver upon the nervous system. For example, a mixture of sound energy falling upon the ears, and through the ears, eventually registering in the brain.

Sensation: Limiting ourselves to the human, the effects of the stimulus upon momentary awareness. These effects may be conveyed verbally. For example, "I hear a rumbling sound increasing in loudness."

Perception: The object or event identified as the *source* of the sensation. For example, "I hear a truck approaching." More generally, the coherence or structuring brought to sensation. The verbal report that there is a truck approaching is presumed to be a fact, and consensus adds to the strength of the presumption that it is a fact.

The Structuralists

The structuralist school was the first to attempt to describe quantitatively how the mind becomes organized. They used the laboratory to work toward a meticulous, introspective examination of consciousness. Despite the fact that they assigned preeminence to the mind, they departed from Plato in their view of the mind's connection to reality. They asserted that reality was neither "inside" nor "outside," but consisted of the *relations* between the two, relations which established how the mind was organized. Hence, the word "psychophysics," which is virtually synonomous with their school.

Although structuralism no·longer exists as a formal enterprise, there are at least three features of this school which remain pertinent to the contemporary psychologist. First, its laboratory techniques remain quite useful in both basic and applied research. Second, its cosmological orientation through Fechner (its chief originator) is downright intriguing, and is quite relevant to modern Western interest in meditative practices, and—more broadly—to Eastern views of human nature. And third, its relation to modern interpretations of consciousness, and perhaps even to the current field of cognitive psychology, is yet to be definitely evaluated.

Definitions of Consciousness and Mind

To pursue our study of structuralism, we require working definitions of both consciousness and mind. We can borrow those of Titchener, the last of the great structuralists:

Consciousness is the sum of mental processes which make up . . . experience *now*; it is the mind of any given 'present' time.

Mind [is] nothing more than the whole sum of mental processes experienced in a single lifetime.[9]

Phrased somewhat differently, "mind" consists of the total accumulation of a person's sensations, feelings, awareness of his existence, up to his present point in life. "Consciousness" consists of the momentary mental experience at that point.

We need not get bogged down with these Titchenerian definitions. They are given mainly so that we may compare the earlier views of Plato, Descartes, and Kant with those of the principle figures of structuralism.

The Originators and Elaborators of Structuralism

The structuralists proper can be divided into two groups: Weber and Fechner comprise one cluster; and Wundt, Kulpe, and Titchener comprise another. The division is based on how far these individuals extended the methodologies of sensory psychology and psychophysics. The first pair were the *originators*;

the second three were the *elaborators*. All were German except for Titchener, who was born in England and came to teach at Cornell at 25. Weber and Fechner introduced the concept of a just notice-able difference (*jnd* or difference threshold) in sensation. By convention, a *jnd* is specified as either an increase or decrease in level of sensation that is detected midway between chance (50 percent of the time) and certainty (100 percent of the time). Of course, this leaves us with the criterion that 75 percent of the judgments would be "Yes, there is an increase (or a decrease) in level of sensation."

Weber dealt with the question of whether there is a definite mathematical relation between the jnd required for a *change* in sensation, on the one side, and the prerequisite *change* in stimulus value on the other, *regardless of what stimulus value we start with*. The results of his careful investigations with trained observers led to the law that bears his name. Weber's Law states: A stimulus must be increased (or decreased) by a constant fraction of its original value, in order for a sensation to become just noticeably different. The uppermost portion of figure 2.2 shows this law in graphical form.

Fechner was an unusual person. As noted by Gardner Murphy:

Nothing could be more misleading than to study Fechner as a follower of Weber, as if he were simply an echo or a reflected light from the great physiologist . . . he was deeply stirred by the "philosophy of nature," which was dominated by the desire to find a spiritual meaning in all the events of the natural order. . . . The universe, said Fechner, is an organism with articulate parts, living and rejoicing in living. Each of the stars and planets, each stone, each clod of earth, has its organization, and organization means life, and life means soul. Everything is imbued with a consciousness of itself and a response to the things about it. This view . . . |is| as pantheistic as Hinduism. It is a far cry from this to that parallelism which says that mental processes and brain processes go on without relation, like two trains moving on tracks side by side. Fechner was assumed to be a parallelist. But for him the world had become one; the experience which men have as persons is of the very substance of the universe, all of which is throbbing with life and experience. This life

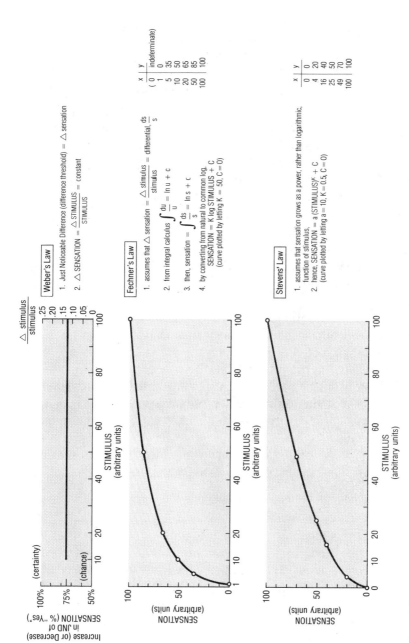

Figure 2.2 Representative curves illustrating Weber's Law, Fechner's Law, and Stevens' Law. In the uppermost panel, the vertical axis on the right serves only to specify the value of Weber's ratio. "Certainty" (the axis on the left) is unrelated to the magnitude of that value, which is constant for any particular sense.

we may, if we choose, study quantitatively; we may study it in the physical laboratory, or in measuring the intensity of sensations.[10]

Fechner was struck by the implications of Weber's Law both as a cosmologist and as a mathematician.

First, as a cosmologist, Fechner could examine in the laboratory the composition of consciousness in humans, by means of their verbal Yes's and No's to changes in sensation. Thereby, he hoped to gain a glimmer of how consciousness was organized in those physical aspects of the universe which did not possess the attribute of speech. In a refined cosmology, organization *itself* represents a form of consciousness. To backtrack a moment: recall that for primeval man, the lack of distinction between biological and nonbiological aspects of the world (or rudimentary cosmology) was based upon the presence of *action* in both. For Fechner, who was much influenced by the sophisticated cosmology of Hinduism and Zen Buddhism, the lack of distinction between the biological and the nonbiological was based upon the presence of *organization* in both. A jug possesses organization, as do the molecules in the glob of clay from which the jug is fashioned, as does the person carrying the jug. Further, the concept of life is incidental to the concept of organization. For the intellectual cosmologist, the fact that the jug possesses organization means that it is just as much "alive," in the sense of organization, as the person carrying the jug.

The second standpoint from which Fechner regarded Weber's Law was as a mathematician. By treating

$$\frac{\triangle \text{ stimulus}}{\text{stimulus}}$$

as a differential $|ds|$ and then by integrating the differential, he could describe how successively accumulating values of sensation were mathematically related to growth in value of any type of stimulus. By assuming two numbers for the constants of integration, a theoretical sensation curve—logarithmic in form—is shown in the middle panel of figure 2.2.[11] What an exciting prospect! What an elegant rationale for obtaining difference thresholds (or Weber ratios) for every one of what Tichener eventually catalogued as over 40,000 fundamental sensations comprising consciousness.[12] Through the calculus of integration, a *jnd* of sensation obtained *mathematical* meaning, it became conceptually responsible for every one of the Fechnerian logarithmic curves.

There was just one problem with the log plot—it is impossible for sensation to go through any stimulus value of *less* than 1 unit since the log of 1 is already 0. That mathematical fact sets an arbitrary limit on where the *absolute* threshold for any sensation might appear. Some theoreticians shrugged this off; for others, it became a matter of major concern.

Using different assumptions (ones hardly tainted with cosmology or with the treatment of the *jnd* as a differential), S. S. Stevens proposed that a power equation more accurately related sensation to stimulus. The problem of the absolute threshold disappeared, because a stimulus value of 0, if raised to any power, remains at 0. A representative curve is shown in the lowermost panel of figure 2.2. The constants were deliberately selected to generate a curve whose form is roughly similar to the Fechnerian curve. The point is that laboratory studies generally yield data which can be fitted either by Fechner's Law or by Stevens' Law. As George Miller noted in his *Mathematics and Psychology*, the distinction between the two laws is "not easily submitted to experimental test."[13]

Challenges to Fechnerian Structuralism, and Some Newer Ideas of Consciousness

We have seen that despite the diverse combination of structuralism's cosmology, mathematics, and science, its psychophysical methodology took hold. Ironically, these very techniques were quickly used to challenge Fechner's assumptions regarding consciousness, thought, and mind.

We will first survey the challenges brought to Fechner's position by Wundt, Kulpe, and Titchener. The philosophical and laboratory pressure they generated was so successful in refuting Fechnerian ideas of consciousness, that the study of consciousness, thought, and mind lay dormant until its relatively recent revival by cognitive psychology. For a considerable period of time, first functionalism, and then the more strident behaviorism, dominated psychology.

We will then comment briefly on more recent understandings of the study of consciousness, those offered by Langfeld, Tart, and Hilgard.

Wundt: Parallelism

Perhaps Wundt's main intellectual contribution was to separate psychology from Fechner's mysticism. He established experimental psychology as a respectable science, based upon physics and physiology. Nonetheless, the specific subject matter of psychology remained for him the study of immediate experience or consciousness, as it had been for Fechner. Wundt expanded the concept of immediate experience to include not only elementary sensations from sensory organs (as in vision and hearing), but also sensations from feeling and volition. However, his formulation and methodology concerning feeling and volition have not gained acceptance. They are now principally of historical rather than scientific interest.

Wundt is known as a parallelist, with the usual explanation of the term being that "He regarded the mind and body as parallel but not interacting systems." [14] While that statement separates Wundt from Descartes's spiritual interactionism, such a description of parallelism hardly does justice to Wundt's position. We must remember that Wundt was a positivist; his parallelism must be understood in that light. For him, a stimulus simultaneously triggered both a neurological event *and* an experiential event, or sensation. Although the neurological event was *necessary* to the mental, the consequences of each event could be studied independently of the other within distinctly separate frames of reference: the physiological or the psychological. Thus, the Helmholtz Doctrine (consciousness and mind are reducible to materialistic variables) is not a constraint upon the examination of consciousness. It is in this way that parallelism attains positivistic meaning. But there is an important proviso: it is that the cardinal *psychological* assumption of structuralism must be met; namely, that an unconfounded analysis of immediate experience is possible. Here it is crucial to recall the key distinction between immediate and mediate experience. The former assumes that sensations *can* be isolated from their context, that one can isolate a sound increasing in loudness, from the fact that the source of the sound is an approaching truck. The mediate position is skeptical that such a dissociation is possible. We shall return to this critical issue in discussing Titchener's "Core-Context Theory of Meaning."

Kulpe: Imageless Thought

Although Wundt and Titchener gave fairly similar and specific definitions of consciousness and mind, neither was so diligent in defining *thought*. In the first place, they held that psychology was concerned with immediate experience, not with cognition, as the higher mental activities were not accessible through study. In the second place, "mind," or the accumulation of a lifetime of "immediate experiences," seemed to them to dispose of thought: thought was just an aspect of the mind. In the third place, any function of thought that we would ordinarily include under the term "reasoning," was deliberately excluded from the laboratory as constituting a "higher mental function," and therefore not the proper subject matter of psychology. Their data was based upon hundreds of trials with subjects (often themselves) trained to discount the intrusion of thought. Such an attitude seems strange to some of us, especially in these days of an earnest cognitive psychology. However, we need remember that all seekers after truth, contemporary as well as past, fall victim to their own paradigms.

Although Kulpe is remembered for having demonstrated that thought could occur without sensations or images of them ("images" are retained and recalled sensations), his protestation was *not* crucial to structuralism, since thought in general had been excluded from psychology's subject matter. What *was* important however, was a finding concerning judgments of lifted weights made by one of Kulpe's students, Karl Marbe. The finding challenged the axiom that sensations (or images of them) were necessarily utilized during the judgment of differences between stimuli. The weight-lifting experiment was then (as it is now) a standard experiment in practically any student's laboratory education. Marbe flouted convention by interrogating his subjects! He found no evidence that the active comparison of sensations entered into their judgments of "heavier" or "lighter." The subjects had no idea as to how they made their judgments, but they were absolutely certain that they did not deliberately compare sensations.

Wundt and Titchener reacted by vigorously condemning the experimental procedures of Kulpe. His unorthodox introspective techniques were considered invalid, in that the questioning of subjects may have changed their attitudes or motivation. As it turned out, Kulpe and his student were, of course, right.

Titchener: Core-Context Theory of Meaning
His dispute with Kulpe notwithstanding, as Titchener grew older, his confidence in the purity of introspective procedures waned. He found that despite the experimenter's and the subject's striving for objectivity, the *context* in which the stimuli were presented gave *meaning* to the stimuli. The meaning, in turn, influenced the way in which the *core* of ostensibly "pure" elementary sensations was reported. The sensation of "greenness" is dependent not only upon spectral composition, but also upon whether the spectral dimensions are presented in the context of grass, or of a leaf.

Initially, this supposed "mistake" in identifying sensations was termed "stimulus error," and then "object error." Gradually, however, Titchener abandoned his hope that sensations could ever be reported independently of context or meaning. Meanwhile, he made an important contribution to psychology. Titchener pointed out that the chronologically *first* context in which sensations were interpreted is not *external* to the individual. Instead, these sensations involve the organism's production of kinesthetic stimuli through his own bodily movements. Depending upon whether the kinesthetic stimuli originate in feedback from general bodily orientation, from specific approach, or from specific withdrawal (three dissimilar contexts), the *same* sensations will be differently interpreted.[15] The portion of Titchener's theorizing pertaining to kinesthesis ties in closely with ideas expressed by Langfeld in his "A Response Interpretation of Consciousness."

The Contributions of Langfeld, Tart, and Hilgard

Langfeld: Efferent Feedback

Once it is recognized that the developmentally prior context in which sensations arise is kinesthetic in origin, then the idea of consciousness as being composed of elementary sensations must take that fact into account. The concept of consciousness must be expanded to include *efference*; it can no longer be limited to the excitation of sensory organs, and the *afference* which brings that excitation to the brain. Consciousness is a closed-loop matter.

Princeton's Langfeld made this point through the way he defined response: "Response means, as here used, response of the organism. In the response is included the entire afferent-efferent system and the receptors, affectors, and central connecting paths."

He went on to comment on the parallelistic implications of neurological systems for a *psychological* understanding of consciousness: "One of the consequences of the identification of consciousness with the efferent as well as the afferent nervous process is that such a theory runs counter to the most widely accepted view of the localization of the mind in the brain, a view which has been held with few exceptions since the early days of philosophical speculation."[16]

His reminder that mind is not solely a function of the brain is as pertinent today as when it was first issued a half-century ago.

Tart: Altered States of Consciousness

Langfeld's attempt to broaden our concept of consciousness is a psychophysiological expansion of the conventional view that consciousness is primarily a function of the brain. Tart went much further.[17] He suggested that our view of consciousness and of reality itself is unduly constrained by the routine paradigms we live by as "normal" people and as scientists. He wondered whether it is possible for scientists in a conventional state of consciousness and of reality, to agree upon the changes in logic that govern the actions of persons in another state of consciousness, since there may be too much of a paradigm shift to permit consensual validation. He framed three plain questions, and implied answers to each: (1) Can two or more persons undergo a similar change in state of consciousness (for example, Zen meditation), return to the normal state, and then agree upon the qualitative nature of the experience that they have undergone? Tart's answer is Yes, allowing for individual differences, which are present even in the so-called "normal" state. (2) Can behavioral scientists in a normal state of consciousness intervene during Zen meditation in others, and then agree that they have obtained the same kinds of perceptual, conditioning, or cognitive data? Here again, Tart's answer is Yes. (3) Can behavioral scientists enter into an altered state of consciousness *similar to that of their subjects*, obtain data, return to the normal state, and then evaluate their data in conventional, positivistic terminology, with any hope of attaining consensual validity? Here, Tart is frank enough to say he does not know. However, he believes that it is possible to find out, without mysticism. He warns, however, that the scientists and subjects will have to be especially well-trained for these investigations—an observation reminiscent of the structuralists' view of how introspective methods attain validity.

Hilgard: Consciousness in Contemporary Psychology

It was mentioned earlier that thought and reason were set aside not only by the structuralists, but also by the yet-to-come behaviorists. During the past few years, associationistic behaviorism has yielded part of the sectarian battleground to non-associationistic cognitive psychology. A renewal of interest in consciousness resulted.

Ernest G. Hilgard has pointed out that:

The new interest in consciousness has produced a wave of writing on the mind-body problem, with each of the classical proposals favored by individual writers, even though every writer believes that new arguments or aspects have been contributed to the discussion. . . . My reaction is that psychologists and physiologists have to be modest in the face of this problem that has baffled the best philosophical minds for centuries.[18]

To keep the topics of consciousness, thought, and mind within psychology in the future, and to prevent another rejection, Stanford's Hilgard has urged that we adopt a "spirit of critical realism," an attitude of inquiry that employs two different types of scientific discourse. The position is described as follows:

There are conscious facts and events that can be shared through communication with others like ourselves, and there are physical events that can be observed or recorded on instruments, and the records then observed and reflected upon. Neither of these sets of facts produces infallible data, for data, if accurate, may be incomplete, and inferences, regardless of how the data are obtained, may be faulty. It is the task of the scientist to use the most available techniques for verification of the data base and for validation of the inferences from these data. The position here recommended is sometimes called a double-language theory that need not commit itself regarding ultimates.[19]

Recapitulation

Beginning with early man's first gropings toward mind-body dualism, we have whisked through a sampling of several philosophical positions concerning mind, and sketched briefly structuralism's scientific attempts to come to grips with consciousness and mind. We have learned that both ancients and moderns were "right"—up to a certain point. It was only when claims were made for the existence of all-inclusive models that problems arose. New attempts inevitably followed in order to resolve the discrepancies by way of still other models. These, in turn, were found fallible, and the cycle repeated itself. Such is characteristic not only of structuralism, but of all forms of psychological inquiry; indeed, of all philosophy and science.

In this context, Hilgard encourages an attitude of temperateness, one that avoids ultimates. Years earlier, Abraham Maslow was even more direct in expressing his concern for the way psychologists approach understanding: "Unfortunately, too many psychologists are not humble, but are, rather, swollen with little knowledge." [20]

As we go on to examine the strengths and weaknesses of other psychological systems, we shall time and again find cause to recognize the wisdom of these words.

3 Functionalism: Goal-Direction, Purpose, Feedback Theory, and Feedback Research

There are four objectives to this chapter: first, to define functionalism; second, to comment on "purpose" as a key concept of functionalism; third, to relate purpose to feedback theory; fourth, to illustrate how feedback theory is expressed in modern research.

Definition of Functionalism

Functionalism is eclectic. Its interests are so broad that functionalism resists designation as a "school" falling within sharply defined theoretical or experimental boundaries. There is no single "functionalism," nor was there ever much of a desire among its leaders that there be one. In describing his own version of functionalism, Columbia's R. S. Woodworth wrote somewhat impatiently that it "does not aspire to be a school. That is the very thing it does not wish to be. Personally, I have always balked on being told, as we have been told at intervals for as long as I can remember, what our marching orders are—what as psychologists we ought to be doing, and what in the divine order of the sciences psychology must be doing."[1]

Nonetheless, we still require some overall definition, one that encompasses the broad concerns of functionalism. Functionalism is the study of psychological processes in general, with emphasis upon their adaptive qualities in particular, as manifested in behavior ranging from inner experience to motor activity. It may be viewed as lying along a continuum, with the narrower schools of structuralism and the yet-to-come behaviorism included as endpoints. Specifically, it includes subject matters as diverse as learning, volition, affect, physiological psychology, developmental psychology, psychophysics—practically everything from nerve cell to neurosis. In short, except for its emphasis upon purposiveness, functionalism is hardly distinguishable from contemporary psychology.

Functionalism was strongly influenced by Charles Darwin's work. Discovery of the propensity of organisms to adapt to the environment led to questions concerning the circumstances under which adaptation occurred. These questions were asked as eagerly by psychologists as they were by biologists. The reason is straightforward. Individual organisms do not survive long enough to produce progeny unless they are first capable of learning to contend with the environment, with each other, and with other species. Natural selection includes the organisms's ability to learn, or to adapt to circumstances, during the course of its life.

William James and Purposivism

William James, one of America's greatest psychologists, held that the ability to adapt to the demands of the world was revealed by the presence of goal-directed behavior. The outward manifestation of goal-directed behavior, in turn, permitted the inference of purpose. And purposiveness was so characteristic a trait of biological organisms that Harvard's James urged its use as a criterion for distinguishing between living and nonliving entities.

He set the tone in his *The Principles of Psychology* (1890):

If some iron filings be sprinkled on a table and a magnet brought near them, they will fly through the air for a certain distance and stick to its surface. A savage seeing the phenomenon explains it as the result of an attraction or love between the magnet and the filings. But let a card cover the poles of the magnet, and the filings will press forever against its surface without its ever occurring to them to pass around its sides and thus come into more direct contact with the object of their love. . . .

If now we pass from such actions as these to those of living things, we notice a striking difference. Romeo wants Juliet as the filings want the magnet; and if no obstacles intervene he moves towards her by as straight a line as they. But Romeo and Juliet, if a wall be built between them, do not remain idiotically pressing their faces against its opposite sides like the magnet and the filings with the card. Romeo soon finds a circuitous way, by scaling the wall or otherwise, of touching Juliet's lips directly. With the filings the path is fixed; whether it reaches the end depends on accidents. With the lover it is the end which is fixed, the path may be modified indefinitely. . . .

The pursuance of future ends and the choice of means for their attainment are thus the mark and criterion of the presence of mentality in a phenomenon. We all use this test to discriminate between an intelligent and a mechanical performance.[2]

James asserted poetically that from the savage's personal experience with the affect attendant upon two creatures drawing themselves together, the savage projects love between the magnet and the filings. The civilized person presumably knows better, and avoids animism by distinguishing between living and nonliving types of matter. James' criterion for establishing this distinction is that of purposiveness. He infers purposiveness from goal-directed behavior. More precisely, he uses observable *changes* in goal-directed behavior as a criterion for distinguishing between living and nonliving things.

Before examining the validity of James's position, we can sharpen the functionalist meaning of purposivism by reviewing McDougall's elaboration of the concept.

McDougall and Purposivism

The British-born Harvard psychologist William Mc-Dougall expanded on James's reasoning by describing seven ways to infer purposiveness from an animal's behavior:

1. Initiation of activity without any obvious external stimulus
2. Persistence of action independently of whatever stimulus may have initiated it
3. Variation in the direction of persistent activity
4. End of activity with goal achievement
5. Readiness or preparation for new activity
6. Improvement in performance through practice
7. The entire organism is involved, not just isolated reflexes[3]

Within the limits of ordinary experience, James and McDougall are convincing. They distinguished between living and nonliving systems on the basis of the presence of purposiveness in the former, and they suggested criteria by means of which purposiveness may be inferred. Their major criterion is the adjustment of action in such manner as to attain a goal. With the advent of cybernetics, however, the salience of this criterion has diminished.

Cybernetics and Purposivism

Cybernetics deals with self-regulating systems. The word derives from the Greek "kybernetes," meaning steersman. The logic of James's and McDougall's argument must confront the fact that nonliving systems of the servomechanism variety display changes in goal-directed behavior. A single example suffices to make the point: A "smart" surface-to-air missile can propel itself upon detecting a target, and—once on its way—keep changing its position in accordance with the evasive action taken by the target. It can even "learn" to take advantage of any regularities in the target's evasive path.

Does the hunting behavior of the missile permit us to infer that it possesses "purpose?" The founders of cybernetics attempted to deal with this question about forty years ago. Norbert Wiener and others implicitly recognized the limitations of the James-McDougall position, and suggested the reason for them. They stated, "The basis of the concept of purpose is the *awareness* of 'voluntary activity.'"[4] Regardless of the merits of their suggestion, we seem to be forced back to metaphysical dispute concerning the nature of consciousness. However, the issues involved will be clarified if we look more carefully at the very concept of "self-regulating system."

The *idea* of self-regulating systems has been part of the human being's intellectual functioning for ages past. As noted by Ernest Nagel, "Automatic control is not a new thing in the world. Self-regulative mechanisms are an inherent feature of innumerable processes in nature, living and nonliving."[5] For example, the Hindu philosophers conceive of a Harmonious Universe, with the action of each portion influencing all other portions. However, the cosmos cannot be considered harmonious unless each part is capable of being sensitive to *changes* in each and every other component of the universe. In modern language, we would say that every part of such a universe provides *feedback* to every other part. Usually this feedback is of the kind termed "negative," because it acts to *reduce* discrepancies between the activity of the different parts of the universe. ("Positive" feedback *increases* discrepancies. Unless otherwise qualified, "feedback" generally implies negative feedback.)

The use of the word feedback may cultivate a comfortable feeling of consensual understanding, but the understanding might well be superficial. Little will be contributed to scientific knowledge unless the concept of feedback itself is used with the same care and precision as that employed by the engineers, scientists, and mathematicians who founded the field of cybernetics. The warning is important for two reasons. For one, it makes no difference from the point of view of systems theory whether a self-regulating system, as a *system*, is comprised of living or engineered components, or a mixture of both. *The equations remain the same,* as do the definitions of the types of feedback involved. The mathematical steering functions performed by a pilot flying an aircraft are amenable to the same specifications as those of an electromechanical device (automatic pilot), otherwise the servo-mechanism could not even be designed.

For another, we need to be fairly circumspect in our use of the word feedback, because it has become something of a jargony, "you-know-what-I-mean," expression. The techniques and concepts of systems analysis—as employed by economists, physiologists, environmentalists, social psychologists, clinical psychologists, experimental psychologists, and others—can be quite productive, provided they retain their authentic meanings. As observed elsewhere,

the servo-model as a way of regarding phenomena lends itself to pseudo-explanations, in the sense of labeling. It is difficult to resist the tendency to describe old problems in new terms and to believe that the old problems have thereby been solved. To describe . . . "libido" as negative feedback and "superego" as positive feedback merely adds two more labels to an already overworked jargon. The specific activity of neither the practitioner nor the researcher is changed one iota as a result of the change in labels.[6]

We must remember that the language in which the ideas and analyses of systems theory is expressed remains tied to servo-mechanism concepts. First, we should consider at what point the logical extension from electromechanical systems becomes a *misleading,* metamorphical extension to other systems. That is to say, we must determine when the concepts originally derived from electromechanical systems can be used in biological, social, or other systems, without doing violence to their original meaning. Metaphors are an inherent part of science, but unless used properly can make for poor science, as well as poor poetry. Second, we should consider when even the *appropriately* selected metaphor ceases to retain and to convey the original meaning, and becomes a distortion of the original.

We can undertake these considerations only by gaining a firm grasp of the feedback language from which systems theory was developed. The language referred to is one that describes adaptive processes. Adaptation, the central concern of functionalism, cannot be fully understood independently of feedback terminology and systems analysis.

Open-loop Feedback Systems

We begin by distinguishing between open- and closed-loop systems. An open-loop system provides feedback after a response; it does not yield feedback *concurrently* with the response of the system. Thus, it is not capable of self-regulation during the course of any *single* act. It is synonymous with a "ballistic" response, as exemplified by a frog striking with its tongue at a fly, or a hunter firing a shotgun at a rabbit. Once a response is initiated, no further changes can be made. The action is committed, even if it might be faulty. If the target changes position during the response, neither the frog nor the hunter can do anything about it. *After* a particular act is completed, the system may receive signals indicating a "hit" or "miss" ("correct" or "incorrect"), and modify accordingly the *next* response. The system is specified as being "open-loop," because of the absence of *concurrent* feedback during the execution of any single response.

Closed-loop Feedback Systems

There are two types of closed-loop feedback systems, discontinuous and continuous. The discontinuous variety is either entirely "on" or "off." There are no gradations between full output and zero output. This type of system is illustrated in figure 3.1, which describes the way the temperature of a room is commonly controlled. The four main component-functions of this—and all *other*—closed-loop systems are shown in the headings above each box. The first function, "Sampling of Input & Output Information," is served through the concurrent monitoring of both the

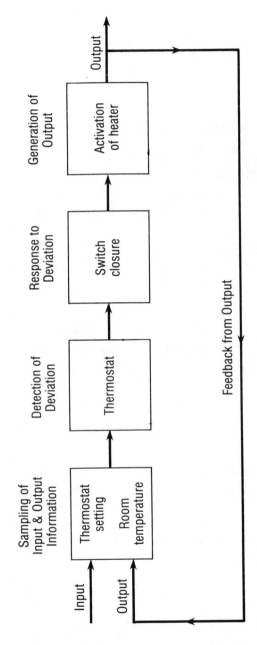

Figure 3.1 Discontinuous closed-loop feedback system: regulating room temperature.

manual setting placed on the thermostat (Input), and the actual temperature in the room (Output). The fact that the thermostat is sensitive to changes in information all the time, and not merely after a response, distinguishes the discontinuous closed-loop system from the open-loop system. The second function, "Detection of Deviation," is enabled by the construction and wiring of the thermostat. If the manual setting is made higher than the room temperature, the switch is closed (third function, "Response to Deviation"). Once the switch is closed, a heater is activated. The heat energy produced in the room (fourth function, "Generation of Output"), feeds back as room temperature, and is continuously sampled. When the discrepancy (the engineering term is "error") between Input and Output is detected as having been removed, the switch is again opened, and the heater is turned off.

The explanation thus far may leave the impression that the discontinuous system is sensitive to the *slightest* input-output discrepancy. However, we know from our own experience with such systems that the thermostat requires a specific, fixed amount of discrepancy between input and output before the error can be detected. Hence, there is a "lag-time" produced by the interval taken for the error to increase until it is large enough to be detected. The presence of this lag-time invites undershoots, as the room becomes colder than would be expected based upon the setting placed on the thermostat. The same holds true in the opposite direction. The heater stays on for a longer period than is necessary (overshoots), because a "discrepancy" of zero is too small to be detected. Attempts to modify the thermostat to minimize the discrepancy (and therefore the time) required for detection, run into the problem of the heater frequently switching from on (full output), to off (zero output). The system thus wastefully oscillates about the desired temperature. This dilemma (lag-time vs. oscillation) is inherent to discontinuous systems, and can be resolved only through engineering compromise.

The continuous closed-loop feedback system is more sophisticated. It is called "continuous" because *gradations* of correction are possible. The system can detect and respond not only to the magnitude of the discrepancy between input and output. It

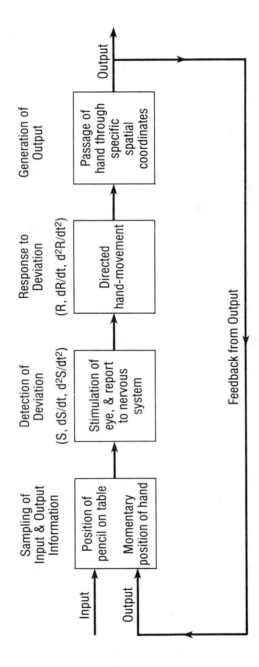

Figure 3.2 Continuous closed-loop system: Wiener's pencil.

can also respond to the first and second and higher time derivatives of error. (The first time derivative is "rate"; the second time derivative is "acceleration.") The problem of lag-time is almost eliminated. The tendency to overshoot and undershoot the "goal" is considerably lessened. Figure 3.2, "Wiener's Pencil," shows these time derivatives, and describes how such a system operates. "S" designates the momentary visual space between hand and pencil; "R", the momentary motor response (limb displacement) required to close the distance between hand and pencil. The figure illustrates the following excerpt from Norbert Wiener's epoch-making book, *Cybernetics*:

Now suppose that I pick up a lead-pencil . . . our motion proceeds in such a way that we may say roughly that the amount by which the pencil is not yet picked up is decreased at each stage. . . .

To perform an action in such a manner, there must be a report to the nervous system, conscious, or unconscious, of the amount by which we have failed to pick the pencil up at each instant.[7]

Note that the example involves a living system, but this is not a requirement (recall the surface-to-air missile). Further, the pencil need not be in a fixed position on the table. It could move about, as it would were the table on a ship at sea.

Figure 3.3, "Driving a car," illustrates both of these features. First, it represents a combined living and nonliving (or man-machine) system. Second, the input changes continuously, unless one were driving on a perfectly straight road.

Interim Consolidation and Some Reflections

We will now review the contents of the chapter thus far, and reflect briefly upon them.

The keystone of functionalism is its concern with adaptive processes, particularly as manifested in goal-direction. From observation of goal-directed behavior, the investigator infers purpose. Equally important, early functionalists (James and

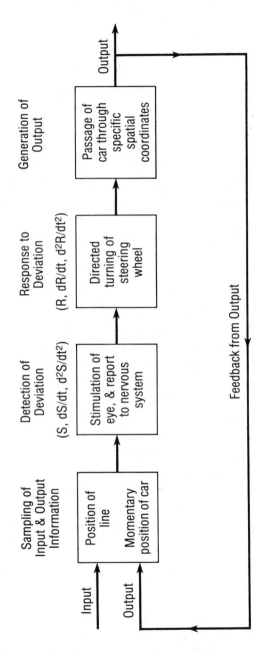

Figure 3.3 Continuous closed-loop feedback system: driving a car.

McDougall) used modifications in such behavior as a criterion for distinguishing between living and nonliving systems. With the advent of cybernetics, however, scientists were forced to reconsider ancient metaphysical disputes concerning the presence of purposiveness within the universe.

We cannot settle metaphysical issues. We can only note that it is once again no longer obvious that the concept of purpose can be limited to living systems. It will become even more enigmatic a problem in the future, as computers and robots that "learn" become more prevalent.

Scientists tend to become uncomfortable with the idea of purposivity for still another reason. Closed-loop systems invite circular explanations, or a confusion of cause with effect. The quandary is that much of our behavior *is* of a closed-loop variety, and therefore effects *do* become causes. Good science demands that we not be so leery of tautologies as to become paralyzed in the laboratory. We must still do all that we can to be deterministic in research concerning purposive behavior. For example, we should not "in our fear of the telological undertones to the words 'purposivism' and 'functionalism' ignore the evidence that lower forms of life (let alone man himself) can extrapolate in time from the immediate present, based upon cueing information provided by the momentarily changing values of current discriminative stimuli."[8] Organisms can bring the future into the present, as it were, through a combination of *current* peripheral discriminations, central planning, and motor actions. Consistent with this observation is the evidence that the greater the regularity or coherence in the cueing information available, the greater the likelihood that purposiveness—in the sense of *learning to use first and second time-order cues to plan ahead*—will be demonstrated.[9]

"Awareness" need not necessarily accompany extrapolations or integrations in time from time-derivative information. Awareness may well be the basis for the *origin* of the concept of "purpose" in the human being's goal-directed behavior. (Recall the remarks of Norbert Wiener et al. above, as well as the analysis of animism in the first chapter). Yet awareness is not always necessary for human goal attainment. In routine driving by the well-practiced driver, for example, the quality of awareness is often lost. However, the act of driving is nonetheless purposeful; the driver still has a goal or destination. Furthermore, the individual often modifies his behavior to attain a particular objective, and does so without being aware of the modification or the objective.

A final point by way of transition toward considering representative research based upon feedback theory: continuous feedback systems have the ability to detect and to respond not only to the momentary absolute difference between system input and output, but also to the first and second time-derivatives of the discrepancy. The figures entitled "Wiener's pencil" and "Driving a car" called attention to changes in space with respect to time, as pertinent examples. Once the importance of detecting and responding to time-derivatives of space is recognized, we make philosophical contact with Kant, and research contact with Piaget. In so doing, we bring together the psychophysics of structuralism, and the goal-directedness of functionalism.

Kant, Piaget, and the Discrimination of Differences in Target Velocity

Both Kant and Piaget held that certain core ideas, such as space and time, are innate. They are innate in the sense that these ideas will begin to emerge during the course of normal development, regardless of the special character of the individual's experiences during childhood. Moreover, these fundamental ideas are not fixed once they emerge, but change as a consequence of apperceptions (Kant) or conceptions (Piaget). ("Apperception" has been defined as "the ability to develop a new perception, through assimilating current knowledge and experience with previous knowledge and experience"; see chapter 2.) "Conception" is quite similar to apperception, with the main difference being that conception includes physiological-maturational factors. Kant's emphasis was upon reason and philosophy; Piaget's was upon child development and research.

Of special interest in the context of this chapter is Piaget's argument that the idea of *velocity*, as conveyed by observing a moving object, is an especially difficult conception for the child to acquire. This is the case because the conception of velocity rests upon combining two prior, basic ideas—those of spatial traverse and of elapsed time. It is for this reason that the two- to seven-year-old child is confused when making judgments involving an object's movement. This is especially evident when moving objects are used as visual targets for testing the ability to discriminate between greater and lesser velocities. The child's difficulty is so striking that Piaget employed velocity discrimination as a major criterion for separating the preoperational from the operational child. The latter *is* capable of conceptualizing ideas of movement.[10] Put more strongly, Piaget believed that it was *impossible* for the preoperational child to organize concurrently changes in space and time. The way he tested his hypothesis is succinctly described by Phillips.[11] (Figure 3.4 assists in following his description of the experiment.) "For example, if two objects move simultaneously—i.e., if they start simultaneously and stop simultaneously—but at different velocities, the child will deny their simultaneity of movement. To him, each moving object has a different 'time,' and one that is a function of the *spatial* features of the display."

In technical language, the display used by Piaget is known as "isochronal," because the two objects in traverse are presented for equal amounts of time.[12] Such being the case, it is obvious that the faster of the two targets will cover the greater distance. But this is not apparent to the preoperational child. He reorganizes the configuration, and *denies* equality of time. The fact that Object B (see figure 3.4) travels a longer distance is attributed to what "must" be an increase in the *duration* of the movement. The preoperational child cannot concurrently synthesize space and time to provide an independent and stable conception of velocity that is directly perceived as such. The conception that he has breaks down into the prior dominance of space and time considered separately. The faster target becomes "equal" in velocity to the slower target. A pseudo-difference in time "explains" the greater distance covered by the faster target.

After approximately seven years of age, human beings

Display

Object A · · · · ▷

Object B · · · · ▷ · · · · ▷

Actual Configuration

$$\text{Velocity A} = \frac{\text{space 1}}{\text{time}}$$
$$\text{(slower)} \qquad \text{(constant)}$$

$$\text{Velocity B} = \frac{\text{space 2}}{\text{time}}$$
$$\text{(faster)} \qquad \text{(constant)}$$

Preoperational Child's Conception

$$\text{Velocity A} = \frac{\text{space 1}}{\text{time}}$$
$$\text{("constant")} \qquad \text{("shorter")}$$

$$\text{Velocity B} = \frac{\text{space 2}}{\text{time}}$$
$$\text{("constant")} \qquad \text{("longer")}$$

Figure 3.4 Preoperational child's conception of isochronal target velocity.

no longer have difficulty in making visual velocity discriminations based upon isochronal displays. More importantly, they can successfully put together an object's traverse through some *quasi-random combination* of space and time, perceive directly the resulting synthesis of velocity, and compare it with another quasi-random combination.[13]

Thus far, we have discussed research that emphasizes the visual discrimination of target velocity, and differences between such velocities. However, we must recognize that the perception of target velocity or the change in spatial traverse with respect to time (ds/dt), is a narrow matter compared with the wider inquiry into the perception of changing exteroceptive stimuli in general. These dynamic stimuli include lines, forms, contours, brightnesses, loudnesses—any type of stimulus flux that can be detected and responded to.[14]

The foregoing is equally germane to research bearing upon proprioceptive stimuli. (Following Sherrington, the terms "proprioceptive" and "kinesthetic" are here used interchangeably.) These internal cues are often of response origin, i.e., response-produced feedback stimuli. They are contained in R, dR/dt, and d^2R/dt^2 (see figures 3.2 and 3.3). It may seem somewhat unusual at first to describe responses as if they were "stimuli." But such is the character of response-produced motor feedback, at least before motor programs develop. The importance of regarding these responses as possessors of stimulus content is considered more fully in the chapters on American Behaviorism and Russian Dialectical-Materialist Psychology. For the present, we need but recognize that figures 3.2 and 3.3 involve "tracking" behavior, and extract the idea that such behavior is representative of everyday visual-motor organization.

Tracking Behavior as a Paradigm for Relating Cognition and Performance

The idea is hardly new. Cybernetics developed in large measure as a consequence of World War II having brought together engineers, mathematicians, and psychologists. Their mission was to provide a theoretical framework, now known as control theory, for the solution of problems stemming from the use of the human being as error detector and error corrector in man-machine systems.[15] Often as not, these functions involved the behavior of an operator watching a cathode ray tube (CRT), and conjointly using a control stick to place and to keep a cursor on a target moving back and forth across the midline of the CRT. This is called "pursuit tracking." The target represents the system's input; the cursor, the output. (In figure 3.3, the target would represent the "Position of line"; and the cursor, the "Momentary position of car." The control stick replaces the steering wheel.) The momentary separation between the two is the error and its time derivatives. The operator's tracking assignment is to affect the generation of output in a manner such as to maintain minimal input-output error.

The temptation was strong to treat the operator as if he were merely a biophysical machine, and some succumbed. Others, such as E. C. Poulton of Cambridge University's Applied Psychology Unit, saw an opportunity to use the tracking situation as a paradigm, whereby the organization of visual-motor information could be studied as a cognitive, as well as a "mechanical," challenge to the operator.[16] The utility of employing the tracking paradigm as a research tool in experiments pertaining to the relations between cognition and human performance has been and continues to be demonstrated.[17] (The connection between cognition and performance is included among the "12 most vital issues" confronting modern cognitive psychology.[18]) However, specific research results can only go so far in influencing scientific and lay opinion. Sometimes the existing culture infiltrates the laboratory, and more directly determines its objectives. In this regard, Posner (1973) has observed: "We have emerged from a period in which all emphasis in theories of thought has been upon verbal or linguistic processes. . . . Probably changes in our general culture . . . have led to increased sympathy for non-verbal processes in thought."[19]

In one nonverbal, cognitive experiment, test-retest

procedures were used to show that there are significant individual differences among college-age subjects in the static and dynamic visual discriminations and motor actions which enter into
visual-motor organization. It was also found that an individual's
excellence in any one of the components entering into visual-motor organization had little to do with his performance in the other
components.[20] In other words, there are both distinctive *within*-in-
dividual differences, and *between*-individual differences. The following brief description of the test-retest experiment is limited to
those visual discriminations which are directly related to the prior
comments concerning Kant and Piaget.

Between- and Within-individual Differences
in Visual Discriminations

Recall that in the Piagetian view the conception of
certain fundamental ideas, such as space, time, and velocity, is
not fixed at birth but changes during the course of development.
If so, then it is possible to entertain the hypothesis that adults
might differ reliably in their ability to discriminate spaces, times,
and velocities, respectively.

In the pertinent experiment, the same 30 subjects (all
of normal vision) were required to render psychophysical judgments on a test-retest basis for differences between: (a) larger and
smaller spatial extents, each distance (horizontal) being marked-
off by two spots of light on a CRT; (b) longer and shorter times,
each time being specified by the duration of a moving target across
a fixed distance; (c) faster and slower target velocities, each velocity being specified from quasi-random combinations of spaces
and times. The subject's performance was assessed on the basis
of percent correct. They arrayed themselves from best to worst in
a reliable test-retest manner for all three configurations, respectively. All test-retest correlations were significant beyond the .01
level of confidence. The test-retest scores were then combined to
yield best estimates of subject proficiency. The cross-correlation

between how the sample of 30 subjects arrayed themselves on judgments of space vs. judgments of time was not significant. Neither were the cross-correlations between space vs. velocity, or time vs. velocity. Thus, the hypothesis concerning adults could not be rejected.

All told, we can safely conclude that between- and within-individual differences are present in quite rudimentary, nonverbal, cognitive ways of organizing space, time, and the synthesis of the two, velocity.[21]

Consolidation

We have come a long way from Romeo and Juliet to feedback theory and research. We have seen that modern technology has questioned whether the demonstration of adaptation (goal direction, purpose), which was once used by functionalists to distinguish between living and nonliving systems, actually does so. We have noted that while this issue is of a metaphysical character, the raising of it has helped bring together the ideas of functionalism and the methodology of structuralism. The sense of the chapter is that cybernetics (or systems theory) helps bridge the two forms of psychological inquiry, thereby enabling each to remain fundamental to modern psychology.

4 Associationism: Philosophical, Experimental, and Clinical Approaches

T his chapter discusses philosophical, experimental, and clinical involvement in the topic of association.

Definitions of Association and Associationism

The word "association" refers to the spatial and/or temporal contiguity of two or more events. As used here, an "event" is an object, a stimulus, a response, an idea, a feeling—anything that is specifiable, either by measurement or through verbal report. "Associationism" refers to the systematic formulations proposed to describe the psychological consequences attendant upon experiencing the contiguity of events. These formulations fall into three main categories: philosophical, experimental, and clinical. Philosophical concern goes back at least as far as Aristotle and continues to this very day.[1] Experimental inquiry began with Ebbinghaus and Thorndike almost a hundred years ago, and is still quite timely. Apart from its own unique orientation, abnormal psychology's theory and application weaves in and out of the philosophical and experimental approaches right from their beginnings.

Despite the fact that this chapter is entitled "Associationism," and the fact that this term conjures up elementalistic accounts of learning and of perception, the limitations inherent in such connectionistic expositions have long been recognized. The problem of balancing elementalism vs. holism which we encountered in our survey of structuralism and functionalism is no less evident in associationism.

Philosophical Associationism

Descartes's ideas concerning the reflex arc were important to the development of associationism, as well as to structuralism. The mechanical-hydraulic prototype of the reflex arc was associationistic, in the sense that a stimulus automatically evoked a response. One event *necessarily* followed another event. As noted in chapter 2, Descartes's concept of the reflex arc was quite sufficient to account for animal behavior, since animals were considered to be nothing more than biophysical machines. However, the concept had to be expanded in order to account for human behavior. The extension consisted of endowing the human being with a soul that possessed cognitive properties. Through thought, the soul made it possible for the human being to interpret stimuli, render decisions, reach conclusions, and exercise free will in implementing these conclusions. Thus, Descartes pulled together a combination of physiological, religious, and philosophical notions: (1) animals were exclusively machinelike; (2) although some of man's behavior was also reflexive, he was basically rational and capable of free will; (3) such was the case because man possessed a soul.

Was Descartes's position designed to accommodate opposing secular and clerical pressures? Rosenblith argues convincingly to the contrary; specifically, he maintains that Descartes was genuinely interested in cognition per se, even though he assigned this function to the reverential soul.[2] Descartes was truly concerned with those attributes of human behavior which could *not* be reduced to reflexlike associations. He considered these attributes useful as "tests": "Given machines or automata capable of simulating faithfully various human actions . . . , he formulated 'two very certain tests' that would distinguish man from brute or more precisely identify those aspects of man's nature that could not be reduced to that of an automaton. The tests relate to (1) the creative use of language and (2) man's enormously varied repertory of actions."[3]

La Mettrie was an uncompromising materialist. He rejected the religious overtones to Descartes's explanation of the soul's interaction with the body. He anticipated the Helmholtz Doctrine by asserting that complex behavior was not a function of the soul, but was attributable to anatomy and physiology. La Mettrie did so by appealing to holistic principles, rather than to elementalistic associations of any form: "Since all the faculties of the soul depend to such a degree on the proper organization of the brain and of the whole body . . . apparently they are this organization itself. . . . The soul is therefore but an empty word, *of which no one has any idea*, and which an enlightened man should use only to signify the part in us that thinks."[4] His meaning is probably clearer if the phrase in italics is changed to read "of which no one *can* have any idea."

La Mettrie's transcendental religious views were quite radical for his time. His account of the soul was unconventional, in that he did not conceive of it as a separate entity. He was literally forced into exile because he was not an orthodox soul-body dualist. Tremendous pressure exists to conform to strictly interpreted, *reified* dualisms of one particular sort or another, despite the alternatives offered by other religious or philosophical orientations. La Mettrie's views were considered to be heretical.

Across the Channel, John Locke's *An Essay Concerning Humane Understanding* set the course for the British philosophical movement known as empiricism. The following positions were taken as axiomatic. First, all ideas originate directly from sensory experience; they do not arise from pure reason. Second, once ideas are gained by a person, they tend to become associated with each other. Third, thought and knowledge consist of these associations.

Locke proposed that there are two distinct types of associations, "sympathies" and "antipathies." The former includes associations that are natural; the latter refers to associations that are fortuitously acquired and unnatural. As an example of the first category, we might take "desk–chair." As an example of the second category, we can take Locke's own, retaining the English of 1700:

Many children imputing the Pain they endured at School to their Books they were corrected for, so joyn those *Ideas* together, that a Book becomes their Aversion, and they are never reconciled to the study and use of them all their Lives after; and thus Reading becomes a torment to them, which otherwise possibly they might have made the great Pleasure of their Lives. There are Rooms convenient enough, that some Men cannot Study in, and fashions of Vessels, which though never so clean and commodious they cannot Drink out of, and that by reason of some accidental *Ideas* which are annex'd to them, and make them offensive.[5]

The relation of the foregoing passage to modern research in aversive conditioning, and to modern views of educational practice is obvious. Not so apparent is the fact that Locke was also hinting at the psychoanalytic concepts of the preconscious and the unconscious. This is revealed in the paragraph preceding the quoted passage:

There is scarce any one that does not observe something that seems odd to him, and is in itself really Extravagant in the Opinions, Reasonings, and Actions of other Men. The least flaw of this kind, if at all different from his own, every one is quick-sighted enough to espie in another, and will by the Authority of Reason forwardly condemn, though he be guilty of much greater Unreasonableness of his own Tenets and Conduct, which he never perceives, and will very hardly, if at all, be convinced of.[6]

Two further observations need to be made before we pass on to James Mill. First, it does not seem to have been important to Locke that sympathies, just as antipathies, were learned and remembered. What a refreshingly optimistic view of human nature! Locke's vision is not confounded by propositions concerning the *innateness* of morally "good" or "bad" ideas. All ideas originated from sensory experience; it was their connections that were either natural or unnatural, reasonable or unreasonable. Second, it is valuable to remember that Locke was a philosopher, not an experimenter, or a clinician. He based his essay upon observing associations that were already formulated in himself and in others. He started with an established association, deduced the components through a conjectural analysis, and then argued how the formulated association might possibly have been induced or put together. Thus, the same person was involved in both the hypothetical deduction (analysis), and the equally hypothetical induction (synthesis).

The same strategy was used by the other British associationists. James Mill's view of how ideas become associated with each other, thereby yielding thought, was so dependent upon tight linkages that it became known as "mental mechanics." Mill held that thought consisted of trains of associated ideas, usually increasing in complexity. Each such train was initiated by a sensation. He wrote:

Thought succeeds thought; idea follows idea, incessantly. If our senses are awake, we are continually receiving sensations, of the eye, the ear, the touch, and so forth; but not sensations alone. After sensations, ideas are perpetually excited of sensations formerly received; after those ideas, other ideas: and during the whole of our lives, a series of those two states of consciousness, called sensations, and ideas, is constantly going on.[7]

The example he gives to explain what he means is plain and to the point: "I see a horse: that is a sensation. Immediately I think of his master: that is an idea. The idea of his master makes me think of his office; he is a minister of state: that is another idea. The idea of a minister of state makes me think of public affairs; and I am led into a train of political ideas."[8] Just at that moment, his thoughts are interrupted by his hearing the call to dinner. "This is a new sensation, followed by the idea of dinner, and of the company with whom I am to partake it. The sight of the company and of the food are other sensations; these suggest ideas without end; other sensations perpetually intervene, suggesting other ideas; and so the process goes on."[9]

Probably Mill was led to his conclusions by working backwards. In examining the first chain of ideas, he may have started out with "Why am I now thinking of politics?" and conjectured analytically to identify in retrospect the links in the chain of associations which had led to the idea of politics. Having identified them, he then presented a synthesis of these components to provide a description of the progression of thought. Needless to say, there was no independent verification at either stage—analysis or synthesis—of this introspective process.

Mill distinguished between two types of associations, synchronous and successive. The former consisted of associations that were established on the basis of spatial contiguity, or "simultaneous existence" in space. For example, "the various objects in my room, the chairs, the tables, the books, have the synchronous order, or order in space."[10] The objects were all associated because of their proximity to each other. One could look at these commonplace objects in different sequences, the chairs first or the tables first. There was no *inherently mandated*, serial order to the way they were sensed, or to the elapse of time separating the observations. However, successive associations *do* involve serial order and temporal contiguity, or "antecedent and consequent existence." For example, "the sight of the flash from the mortar fired at a distance, the hearing of the report."[11] Because the speed of light is much greater than the speed of sound, there is a physically determined basis both to the antecedent and consequent order in which the events are sensed, and to the time separating the two events. Mill also held that of the two types of associations, the successive is more prevalent than the synchronous. The fact is that events in the world, and our relation to them, tend more to keep changing than to remain static. Further, he noted that the strength of both types of associations is influenced by the vividness (i.e., distinctiveness) of the entering component-events, and by how often these events are paired with each other.

Before passing from Mill the Elder to Mill the Younger, we must note James Mill's own uneasiness lest his views concerning the formation of associations be interpreted too rigidly. He carefully observed the following: "In the successive order of ideas, that which precedes, is sometimes called the suggesting, that which succeeds, the suggested idea; not that any *power* is supposed to reside in the antecedent over the consequent; suggesting, and suggested, mean only antecedent and consequent, with the additional idea, *that such order is not casual, but, to a certain degree, permanent.*"[12] One can detect in the foregoing passage the beginning of a distinction between nonreflexive association leading to a psychological impression of connectedness, and logical inference leading to a conclusion of causality. He prepared the way for his son's A *System of Logic*, a work which sets forth rules whereby an inquirer can examine the nature of the relations between regularly correlated events, and can assess the likelihood that a particular antecedent event is the cause of a consequent event.

John Stuart Mill was in accord with his father's distinction between synchronous and successive types of associations. He did not agree with his assertion that complex ideas were reducible to linkages of individual component ideas, trains of which were initiated by sensations. Nor did he agree with David Hume, who held that "it is a fixed feature of the mind to regard as a *cause* any event which reliably precedes and is always 'conjoined' with another event which the mind then takes to be the *effect*. Indeed, the idea of causality is nothing but this constant conjunction between two events narrowly separated in time."[13] Rather, the son believed that complex ideas were generated in a manner analogous to the chemical process whereby water is formed from the combination of hydrogen and oxygen. Even as water has properties that are quite different from its entering elements, so a complex idea possesses characteristics that transcend its entering components. Clearly, J. S. Mill was anticipating the gestalt dictum that "the whole is different from the sum of its parts." Equally apparent is the relation of his mental chemistry to Titchener's core-context theory of meaning (chapter 2), and to Piaget's finding that the perception of velocity requires more than the preoperational child's ability to organize space and time (chapter 3).

Mill the Younger believed that, once complex ideas are formed, they followed the rules of association, such as synchronicity and succession, laid down by his father. He stated: "It may be remarked, that the general laws of association prevail among these more intricate states of mind, in the same manner as among the simpler ones."[14] The importance of synchronous and successive associations in establishing the psychological impression of relations between events (whether physical or ideational), led J. S. Mill to examine the rules that determine causality. He undertook the task because causality, too, is concerned with the relations between events, but from a logical point of view.

Can a sharp distinction indeed be drawn between the nonreflexive association processes, which yield psychological impressions, and the logical inferences, which indicate causality? The problem was hinted at by Kant. Recall that he suggested that the tendency to seek organization among events was a trait *inborn* in human beings. Inborn or not, how much of this trait rests upon impressions, and how much upon logic? The issue can be sharpened if we look more carefully at the fundamental types of association, the synchronous and successive. James Mill's example of the former rested upon the physical proximity of one event to another (his example was the objects in his room). But how "near" is the required nearness of A to B before an association is formed? Clearly, there are limits to the impression of spatial contiguity. These limits are imposed by the amount of intervening space, by the structure and function of A and B themselves, and by the psychological condition of the observer.

The matter of limits notwithstanding, let us accept that spatial contiguity is responsible for Mill's psychological association of chairs with tables. Now suppose he were to have found a nick in the edge of the table he worked on, and a nick in the armrest of the chair he sat upon, and that these damages to his furniture were not only spatially contiguous, but were at a common height from the floor. A logical inference he might have drawn is that he had inadvertently jostled his chair against the table. However, other possible explanations exist. For example, his maid may have carelessly used her mop against both the chair and the table, striking each at the same height. Thus, starting with an association based upon spatial contiguity, and then noticing a common factor, Mill could have drawn the wrong logical inference, and blamed himself for something that another person had done.

In the case of successive associations, the danger of confusion between psychological impression and logical inference is even greater. Using Mill the Elder's own example, it is readily evident that the association between the sight of a specific gun flash, A, and the subsequent hearing of a particular report, B, does not establish that A was indeed the cause of B. The usefulness of seriality between events as a criterion for assuming causality is limited by the number of concurrent antecedent A's that are known (in this case, seen), let alone those that are unknown (or unseen). The notion of seriality is also limited by the length of time elapsing between the events that enter into the sequence; i.e., temporal contiguity. If the elapsed time is too great, irrelevant flashes may preempt the observer's attention, and be incorrectly identified as the antecedent event. Thus, the true gun may go unrecognized if other flashes intervene before the actually-related consequent sound is heard. Further complications arise from the previously mentioned factors of vividness and frequency of paired events. For example, a larger mortar is more likely to engage our attention because of its brighter flash and louder blast. And a gun that is fired more frequently may be more compelling than one that is fired less often.

J.S. Mill's A *System of Logic* is a remarkable attempt to illuminate the gray area between notions of relationship between events that rest upon psychological impressions, and of those that depend upon logical inference. Additionally, his work enables us to understand why even logical inference can be fallible, despite the best efforts of the inquirer.

He generated several rules or canons whereby logical inferences can be drawn. Among them are procedures now known as the Method of Agreement and the Method of Difference. According to the former, that variable which precedes all instances of a given effect is the causative agent. The logic is illustrated in the accompanying schema:

X, Y, Z → effect
X, Y,   → effect
Y, Z → effect
Therefore, Y is the cause

The Method of Agreement is fallible on both experimental and correlational grounds, since the wrong common factor may be identified. There may be another, unknown variable—the "true" cause—that regularly accompanies Y. The method is also fallible on the even prior grounds that no scientist can possibly examine *all* instances leading to a given effect. One or another type of sampling or replication of presumably representative cases must be employed.

The logic of the Method of Difference is illustrated as follows:

X, Y, Z → effect
X,   Z → absence of effect
Therefore, Y is the cause

The causative agent is that variable which, when present, is followed by the effect; and which, when absent, is not followed by the effect. As with the Method of Agreement, there are two sorts of fallibility inherent in this procedure: (1) Y may be regularly accompanied by some unknown variable, the existence of which is unsuspected; (2) the scientist must draw the line somewhere with regard to the number of times he tests for the presence or absence of the effect, and he may cease replicating too soon.

Must we then give up in despair? Only if we believe that either psychology or logic leads to ultimate truth. If we turn these disciplines into *metaphysics*, then we are using them for purposes beyond their legitimate scope. Despite their fallibility, conclusions of association based upon psychological impressions, and of causality based upon logical inferences, *can* be correct. It depends upon the acumen and judiciousness of the observer or the experimenter, with the caveat that sometimes even the best are wrong.

British philosophers defined the areas of associationism and of causality, and specified the variables and methods of interest, but they did not enter the laboratory. We turn now to those associationists who did, the early experimenters.

Experimental Associationism: Ebbinghaus and Thorndike

Psychological research began with Fechner, the combined mystic-mathematician, who almost single-handedly developed the psychophysical methods. The fundamental subject matter studied was "pure" consciousness, and how it was amalgamated from sensations produced by stimuli. The study of higher mental processes, such as learning and thinking, was deliberately excluded from the fledgling science. It was held that these phenomena went beyond the limits imposed by scientific positivism. Nonetheless, higher properties intruded upon psychological data, and Titchener eventually admitted as much.

Hermann Ebbinghaus wanted to reach out experimentally toward these complex mental functions, and to do so through the study of verbal learning and remembering. But paradoxically, he used the building-block, Fechnerian version of laboratory methodology to conduct his investigations. Thereby, he set an extraordinary constraint on what might be legitimately construed as comprising his proper subject matter. His elementalistic approach became so pure as to require the use of meaningless nonsense syllables in his examination of the acquisition and retention of verbal associations. The resemblance to Fechner's rationale is not coincidental. As noted by Duane Schultz:

Fechner's mathematical approach to psychological phenomena was an exciting disclosure to the young Ebbinghaus, and he resolved to do for the study of memory what Fechner had done for psychophysics, through rigid and systematic measurements. He wanted to apply the experimental method to the higher mental processes and decided, probably as a result of the influence of the British associationists, to make the attempt in the field of memory. . . . Ebbinghaus recognized an inherent difficulty in using prose or poetry. Meanings or associations are already attached to words by those who know the language . . . [he therefore] sought material that would be uniformly unassociated, completely homogeneous, and equally unfamiliar—material with which there could be no past associations.[15]

The nonsense syllables he typically employed were of the form consonant-vowel-consonant, such as "VAD." By means of a memory drum, a list of such syllables can be presented sequentially to the subject. A memory drum is a cylinder which rotates about a horizontal axle, with an electric motor supplying the power, and with switches determining the motor's on-off intervals. The syllables are viewed through a frame in consistent, serial order. There is a brief pause between presentations of successive syllables. The task imposed is that of learning to use the first syllable as a cue or stimulus word for the second syllable, and to anticipate verbally the second syllable before it is actually shown. The appearance of the second syllable then serves both to provide knowledge of results for correctness of the prior response, and to act as a cue for anticipating the next or third syllable. This procedure (formally known as the Method of Anticipation) is followed until the entire list of perhaps ten or more syllables is viewed and responded to, thereby constituting a single trial. The list is assumed to be fully learned when the subject can anticipate all the syllables in the list without a single error, usually to a criterion of two consecutive trials so as to reduce the likelihood of chance success.

Of course, there are variations of this fundamental technique. For example, sometimes the first syllable is used as a starting cue (as described in the foregoing); sometimes even the first syllable is anticipated, with the experimenter saying "Now" as a starting cue—not at all an impossible task for the subject after the first run-through of the list. Using the method of anticipation, Ebbinghaus even experimented with associative learning and remembering of lines of poetry, and satisfied himself that this type of material, although easier to learn and to remember, followed the same general laws of association as were obtained from nonsense syllables. Of course, properties of poetry that are untapped by the memory drum—such as metaphor and creativity of expression—remained unexamined. His independent variables included: (1) the exposure time of each syllable, (2) the time between syllables, (3) the number of syllables, and (4) the time elapsing between original learning and the test for retention. The type of data gathered, as well as the kinds of issues that emerged, are illustrated in figure 4.1, "The Ebbinghaus Approach." The left panel shows that when either nonsense syllables or familiar names are learned in consistent serial order (e.g., by means of a memory drum), it is more difficult to acquire and to retain the items in the middle of the list than those toward either end. One theory advanced to account for this phenomenon holds that interference with, or inhibition from, each item with respect to the other is maximal in the middle of the list. The right panel shows that even though the absolute number of errors is greater for nonsense syllables than for names, the *relative* interference (or inhibition) is about the same for both.

Here we must pause for a moment to realize more fully the implications of Ebbinghaus' contribution. Whereas the philosopher-associationists conjectured about the formation of their own trains of *existing* associations, Ebbinghaus studied the formation of *new* associations, and he did so in the laboratory. Thus,

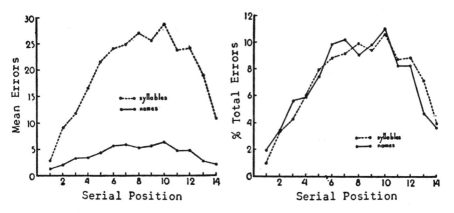

Figure 4.1 The Ebbinghaus Approach. (From R.S. Woodworth and H. Schlosberg, *Experimental Psychology* [1954], revised ed. Copyright © 1938, 1954 by Holt, Rinehart and Winston, Inc. Reprinted by permission of Holt, Rinehart and Winston, CBS College Publishing).

a logical argument for explaining the generation of associations did not rest upon the persuasiveness of a single individual. Other investigators could use Ebbinghaus's experimental procedures, and determine for themselves whether the data were replicable, and form testable hypotheses concerning explanations of the data.

Whereas Ebbinghaus's tactic of studying the formation of new associations was to use human subjects and nonsense syllables, Edward Lee Thorndike's was to use animal subjects and "puzzle boxes." A puzzle box was a cage into which a hungry animal, most often a cat, was placed. The cat could escape through a door which opened when the animal pulled a lever, or a chain, or a wire loop, singly or in some sequence. Upon obtaining its release, the cat was given a morsel of food, and placed again in the cage for another trial. The time-to-escape per trial was recorded. Figure 4.2 is a representative curve, and originally appeared in Thorndike's dissertation.[16]

Thorndike held that

the solution of such a problem by cats and other animals involved the formation of an association between some aspect of the stimulus-situation, such as the wire loop or the wooden lever, with the specific movement that led to door-opening. Further, he argued the stimulus-response relation that finally appeared was obviously influenced by the outcome of this movement. The pleasure experienced by the animal in getting out of the box and to the food served to stamp in the connection between stimulus and response that led to the pleasure. By the same token, stimulus-response connections that did not lead to a pleasurable after-effect were not strengthened, and tended to drop out.[17]

Eventually, Thorndike termed the underlying principle of association the Law of Effect.

But Thorndike was interested in explaining more than just how a cat formed associations. He boldly stated in his dissertation: "our best service has been to show that animal intellection is made up of a lot of specific connections . . . which subserve practical ends directly, and to homologize it with the intellection involved in such human associations as regulate the conduct of a man playing tennis."[18] He was among the first, along

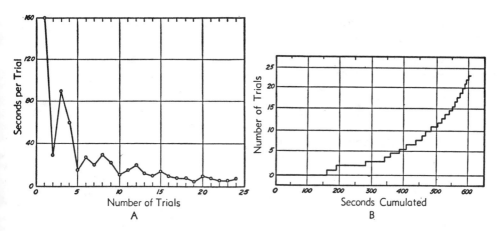

Figure 4.2 The Thorndike Approach. (From R.S. Woodworth and H. Schlosberg, *Experimental Psychology* (1954), revised ed. Copyright © 1938, 1954 by Holt, Rinehart and Winston, Inc. Reprinted by permission of Holt, Rinehart and Winston, CBS College Publishing).

with Pavlov, to argue that animals could be studied in the laboratory in order to illuminate human psychology.

Thorndike's approach stands out for the following additional reasons: (1) His view of stimulus-response connections was one in which stimuli served as *cues*, rather than "goads." His connectionism was a far cry from Cartesian sensory-motor reflexology. (2) His choice of animals, rather than humans, to study associations in puzzle boxes, reflected the joint influence of Darwin's theory of evolution and of functionalism's principle of adaptation through goal-directed behavior. (3) His drawing a parallel between animal and human intellection was not so much a matter of attributing ideational, cognitive properties to the cat, but rather the other way around; namely, to suggest that much of human behavior did not require deliberate thought. (4) His use of food as a reinforcer for the cat's escape from the puzzle box led to the behavioristic premise that reinforcement could retroactively influence the emission of consequent acts. Figure 4.2 is from a classic influential text, and shows the kind of data obtained by Thorndike. It also shows how the data can be replotted to yield cumulative curves of the Skinnerian-behaviorist variety.

The curves are placed in juxtaposition to make the point that Thorndike's connectionism, less its underlying hedonistic overtones, became fundamental to the philosophy of future American behaviorism, which we consider in chapter 6.

Clinical Associationism

Abnormal psychology, like experimental psychology, brought positivism to bear upon the study of associations. The clinician's use of word association tests (such as the Kent-Rosanoff), and of projective tests (such as the Rorschach "ink-blot"), are deterministic extensions of Locke's earlier distinction between natural and unnatural associations. There is a further similarity. As with the British philosophers, clinical-testers deal with *existing* responses, and then work backwards analytically to select the psychological variables that might have induced the responses. Both the Kent-Rosanoff and the Rorschach involve the presentation of stimuli to subjects, and then the tester's analysis of the attendant responses or "free" associations to these stimuli. First, a demonstrational word association test (WAT), and later, a projective situation are provided for illustrative purposes.

As is evident from the demonstrational WAT, the analysis is accomplished by comparing the subject's responses with norms gathered from diverse populations. (If the reader is part of a group, he may want to compare his responses with those of others.)

The principle difference between the two types of tests consists of the amount of structure contained in the stimuli. The verbal stimuli of the WAT are considered to be more structured than the visual stimuli of the Rorschach, and therefore less conducive to sampling a wide range of associations. Nonetheless, the range of associations allowed by verbal stimuli is sufficient to have convinced Jung of the usefulness of this kind of test. He developed one of his own to use for diagnostic purposes, reasoning that departures from conventional norms indicated possible emotional problems. The particular diagnosis made depended upon the *content* of the unique responses, not just their number. Jung was hardly a mental mechanic! He also recorded the time taken to respond to each stimulus-word (i.e., reaction time), and treated long reaction times as evidence indicative of "blocking."

Word association tests are currently used not only by professional clinicians, but also by police and intelligence experts. Charged words, such as the location of a crime or the name of the weapon employed, are included among the routine stimulus words. The content of the responses to these charged words, as well as the time taken to make them, are evaluated.

Considerable research has gone into standardizing the procedure for giving and for evaluating the Rorschach test. A sub-

Table 4.1 Demonstrational Word Association Test

Instructions: Below you will see a list of 20 stimulus words. After each word write the first word that it makes you think of. Start with the first word; look at it; write the word it makes you think of; then go on to the next word. Use only a single word for each response. Do not skip any words. Work rapidly until you have finished all 20 words.

STIMULUS*	RESPONSE
1. Table	_____
2. Dark	_____
3. Music	_____
4. Sickness	_____
5. Man	_____
6. Deep	_____
7. Soft	_____
8. Eating	_____
9. Mountain	_____
10. House	_____
11. Black	_____
12. Mutton	_____
13. Comfort	_____
14. Hand	_____
15. Short	_____
16. Fruit	_____
17. Butterfly	_____
18. Smooth	_____
19. Command	_____
20. Chair	_____

*The first 20 stimulus words of the Kent-Rosanoff Word Association Test

Table 4.1 (cont.)

Instructions: Using your own sense of discretion as to personal privacy, select any of your associations that are illustrative of Locke's "sympathies" or "antipathies." Select any of your associations that are illustrative of James Mill's "synchronous" or "successive" component events.

The Three Most Common Responses to Stimulus Words *

STIMULUS	RESPONSES
1. Table	Chair, Food, Desk
2. Dark	Light, Night, Room
3. Music	Song(s), Note(s), Sound
4. Sickness	Health, Ill, Death
5. Man	Woman(en), Boy, Girl
6. Deep	Shallow, Dark, Water
7. Soft	Hard, Light, Pillow
8. Eating	Food, Drinking, Sleeping
9. Mountain	Hill(s), High, Snow
10. House	Home, Door, Garage
11. Black	White, Dark, Cat
12. Mutton	Lamb, Sheep, Meat
13. Comfort	Chair, Bed, Ease
14. Hand	Foot(ee), Finger(s), Arm
15. Short	Tall, Long, Fat
16. Fruit	Apple, Vegetable, Orange
17. Butterfly	Moth, Insect, Wing(s)
18. Smooth	Rough, Soft, Hard
19. Command	Order, Army, Obey
20. Chair	Table, Sit, Leg(s)

* Based on Russell, W. A., & Jenkins, J. J. The complete Minnesota norms for responses to 100 words from the Kent-Rosanoff Word Association Test, ONR Tech. Rep. 11, 1954 (Contract Number N8 ONR-66216). Because they were obtained so long ago, these norms are not strictly valid, and serve only for demonstrational purposes.

ject is given ink-blot cards one at a time, and instructed to report what he/she sees in each. Broadly speaking, the quality of coherence (or perception) brought to the sensations evoked by the stimuli depends upon the respondee's characteristic interpersonal relations and mode of organizing the world. Responses are classified according to three major categories: (1) *Location,* or the specific portion of the blot that evokes the response (e.g., whole blot, large detail, small detail). (2) *Determinants,* or the specific stimulus attributes selectively attended to (e.g., color, form, apparent movement, shading). (3) *Content,* or the nature of what is perceived (e.g., humans, animals, objects, processes). Why these particular categories? Some rough examples should help make clear the rationale. Consider "Location": whether the respondee uses the whole blot or only a small detail thereof may indicate how he typically organizes life's ambiguous situations. For instance, does he try to get at the total picture, or is he diverted by minor issues? "Determinant": color is presumed to be related to the ways in which affect influences perception and behavior. The expression "He always sees the darker side of things" conveys the idea. If the "Content" of the responses tends to be mainly animals, then it may reflect that the respondee—if an adult—is less than mature in the way he or she relates to other people.

After the responses are classified, the Rorschach expert goes on to consider the interrelations within and among the three major categories of responses. Simply adding up scores is hardly what the Rorschach is about—a holistic, rather than elementalistic, approach is taken.

The principles of projective association apply not only to standardized tests, but extend to works of art that invite a rich variety of interpretations by the viewer. For example, the accompanying photograph of a panel of modern sculpture by Dubuffet can be used to demonstrate the power of projective tests. If two or more people are instructed to look at it with the idea of reporting what they see, and if they write down their responses independently, and then compare them, they will rarely find that their responses are completely identical. Of course, art is meant to be enjoyed for its own sake, without submitting it to psychological scrutiny. But it is also instructive to examine it with the psychologist's eye or ear, as is done in the field of esthetics.

A Concluding Comment

It was noted at the outset of this chapter that "The problem of balancing elementalism vs. holism which we encountered in our survey of structuralism and functionalism is no less

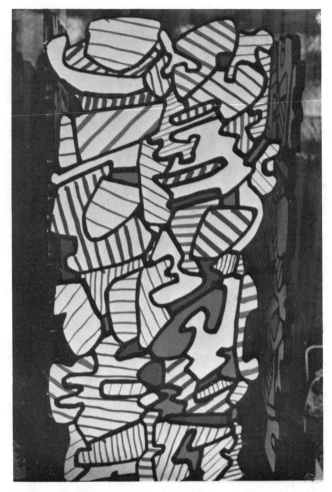

Figure 4.3 Panel of modern sculpture designed by Jean Dubuffet. (From the collection of Rebecca and Joseph Notterman)

evident in associationism." Now that we have scanned the contributions of the philosophical, experimental, and clinical varieties of associationism, it seems that the philosophers and the
clinicians made their compromises, but that the laboratory researchers were more inclined to be elementalists. Perhaps that is
because of the need to specify variables and methodology as pre-

cisely as possible. However, we must remember that experimental psychology has come a long way since Ebbinghaus and Thorndike. As we continue with our examination of forms of psychological inquiry, we shall see that the tension between elementalism and holism has been recognized by researchers, and that the challenge presented by the need for its resolution persists to this day.

5 Russian Dialectical-Materialist Psychology: Prerevolutionary, Revolutionary, and Postrevolutionary Times

Russian ideas concerning the proper subject matter of psychology were markedly influenced by social-political events. The psychology of communist revolutionary (1917) and postrevolutionary times is different from that of prerevolutionary days, and for reasons that were frequently expostulated in terms of communist doctrine, as well as inherent scientific merit. The general objective of this chapter is to sketch the major intertwining social-political, philosophical, theoretical, and experimental features of Russian dialectical-materialist psychology.

Dialectical Materialism: Its Relation to Russian Psychology

"Dialectics" means logical argumentation. Marx utilized Hegelian dialectics, a type which holds that any thesis can be countered by an equally tenable antithesis, and that reasoned consideration of the two opposing points of view will eventually lead to their resolution or synthesis.[1] The synthesis in turn is stated in the form of a new thesis, which leads to its own antithesis, followed by yet another synthesis, and so on. "Materialism" asserts that reality consists of matter; more specifically, matter and its motions.

"Dialectical materialism" is more difficult to define and to grasp than either of its component terms. The problem is that there are two distinct connotations to its meaning. One interpretation is philosophic, the other is economic, even though both views originate in Hegelian dialectics. The *philosophic theory* holds that matter is in a continuous state of transformation. The changes in matter are induced in one of two ways: either (a) by nature— e.g., when clouds are turned into rain, and the resulting water affects a tenuous ecological balance, consequently initiating still further changes; or (b) by man—e.g., when trees are turned into wooden things, and these things are used to make or to obtain a variety of other objects. The availability of these objects enables the production or acquisition of still other items, and so the process of material transformation continues. The *economic* theory affirms that a society containing socio-economic classes inevitably evolves through political thesis, antithesis, synthesis, new thesis, and so on, toward one without classes. Marx and other communist writers believed that the economic version of dialectical materialism necessarily followed from the philosophic. (Equally competent capitalist theoreticians disagree and assert that there is no connection.[2])

Marx's argument for tying the economic theory to the philosophic is the following: whoever owns natural resources (matter) and the means of producing and distributing food and manufactured goods (matter transformed into usable things), directly or indirectly establishes the individual and society's prevailing conception of what is "valuable." In short, there is a dynamic interconnection between things and "value." Private ownership encourages value-concepts which direct production and distribution so as to lead to a selfish, divided society, one that eventually destroys itself. Collective (i.e., state) ownership, however, leads to a cooperative, free society, resting upon the unselfish principle heralded by the slogan "from each according to his ability, to each according to his need."

Because of his emphasis upon the relation between

economic theory and the formation of values, Marx was forced to consider issues which were primarily of a *psychological* character. He tried to show that the supporters of private ownership (whether czarist or capitalist) assumed that peasants or workers could be "programmed" like robots to accept reflexively the particular things they *should* cherish. In contradistinction, Marx and other proponents of communism held that man's behavior was not only reflexive, but also independent. Because of his ability to adapt, his capacity to represent the world ideationally, and his gift for abstract thought, man could *learn* to become both individually purposeful and socially active. It is on these grounds—and not the ones implied by a spontaneous and innate "free will"—that man's behavior can be considered independent.

In his *Philosophical Notebooks* (published posthumously in 1929–30), Lenin sharpened Marx's distinction between the two opposing views of human nature, reflexive and independent. The reflexive was termed "one-way dialectical materialism"; the independent, "two-way dialectical materialism."

One-way dialectical materialism asserts that an understanding of anatomy and physiology (particulary of the brain and central nervous system) is both necessary and sufficient for an understanding of human behavior. Mental life is epiphenomenal, and has no independent influence upon action. In its essentials, one-way dialectical materialism is a restatement of the Helmholtz Doctrine (see chapter 2). Two-way dialectical materialism holds that while a knowledge of the brain's material qualities is necessary for an understanding of human behavior, it is not sufficient. Mentation has its own representative reality (albeit within the constraints mandated by anatomy, physiology, heredity, environment, and past experience), and exerts a perceived autonomous influence on an individual's personal and social behavior.

Prerevolutionary psychology was dominated by one-way dialectical materialism, mainly in the form of I. M. Sechenov's reflexology. Revolutionary psychology tried to come to grips with the political implications of two-way dialectical materialism. K.N. Kornilov's reactology was considered by Soviet authorities and found wanting. Meanwhile, I.P. Pavlov's conditioning research and theory (which preceded and continued through the revolution) was undergoing careful ideological scrutiny, and was eventually decreed to be thoroughly acceptable. Postrevolutionary psychology expanded on conditioning in ways that most Americans are first beginning to comprehend and to relate to their own endeavors. We now look more carefully at each of these stages of Russian psychology.

Prerevolutionary Times

As we know, René Descartes accounted for animal behavior by means of reflex arcs. He maintained that animals are soul-less, biophysical machines. Human beings, because they have souls, possess the capacity to overcome purely materialistic, input-output reflexes. It is for this reason that man can be held morally responsible for his actions.

Ivan Sechenov, a prerevolutionary physiologist, had no place for souls or free will. Unlike Descartes, the *modest* materialist, Sechenov was a *frank* materialist, and he minced no words in presenting his extreme position: "All psychical acts, without exception . . . are developed by means of reflexes . . . all conscious movements (usually called voluntary), inasmuch as they arise from these acts, are reflex in the strictest sense of the word. The question whether voluntary movements are really based upon stimulation of sensory nerves is thereby answered affirmatively."[3]

By "psychical activity," Sechenov implied thoughts, ideas, and imagination, phenomena generally assumed to be autonomous. He asserted that psychical activity is based upon neurological residuals (or traces) of what were originally *overt*, physiological reflexes. The development of a wide repertoire of covert, stimulus-response connections or associations is possible only through purely physiological processes, such as facilitation and inhibition. If we eliminate the physiological assumptions (he offered no conclusive data), Sechenov sounds like a latter-day James Mill.

The Russian scientist was well aware that his bold analysis flew in the face of everyday, personal experience. For instance, how can either *voluntary* movement or *autonomous* thought be said to originate from *direct stimulation* of sensory nerves? His position is best understood if we isolate the three premises upon which it rests. They are:

Premise 1. *Thought is an optico-acoustic trace of a reflex.* In other words, thought consists of visual imagery and hearing one's own internal speech.

Premise 2. *The perceived independence (or free-initiation) of "voluntary" movement and "autonomous" thought is illusory.* So-called voluntary movement and autonomous thought are really initiated directly by external stimuli that go unnoticed. These stimuli go unnoticed for three reasons: (a) They are weak, and are (in today's language) overshadowed. (b) Because they are weak, these stimuli and their attendant indistinct sensations cannot be discerned as initiating a serial order of events. Hence, a connection between these weak stimuli and the ostensibly voluntary movement or autonomous thought fails to be recognized. (c) The time span between the truly initiating (but weak) stimuli and the consequent movement or thought exceeds (in today's language) short-term memory.

Premise 3. *The illusion is maintained through contingencies involving the same thought followed by different acts, or different thoughts followed by the same act.* The perceived independence of voluntary movement and of autonomous thought is abetted not only by overshadowing and by the limits of short-term memory, but also by (in today's language) differential reinforcement, as indicated in the illustration.

Here is an example: I devote my daytime to physiology; but in the evening, while going to bed, it is my habit to think of politics.[4] It happens, of course, that among other political matters I *sometimes* think of the Emperor of China [emphasis added, to underscore the third premise]. This [optico]-acoustic trace becomes associated with the various sensations (muscular, tactile, thermic, etc.) which I experience when lying in bed. It may happen, one day, that owing to fatigue or to the absence of work I lie down on my bed in the daytime; and lo! all of a sudden I notice that

I am thinking of the Emperor of China. People usually say that there is no particular cause for such a visitation; but we see that in the given case it was called forth by the sensations of lying in bed; and now that I have *written* this example, I shall associate the Emperor of China with more vivid sensations, and he will become my frequent guest.[5]

It is easy to see why Ivan Sechenov is considered to be the father of "objective" psychology, of which American behaviorism is an offshoot. And why, too, the intellectuals and scientists of revolutionary Russian found his reflexology overly reductionist for a society that demanded independence of action and thought, without which individual purposivism and social activism would be impossible.

Interestingly, the American philosopher, John Dewey, wrote what is probably the most devasting criticism of reflexology. He said:

We ought to be able to see that the ordinary conception of the reflex arc theory, instead of being a case of plain science, is a survival of the metaphysical dualism, first formulated by Plato, according to which the sensation is an ambiguous dweller on the border land of soul and body, the idea (or central process) is purely psychical, and the act (or movement) purely physical. Thus the reflex arc formulation is neither physical (or physiological) nor psychological; it is a mixed materialistic-spiritualistic assumption.[6]

Revolutionary Times

The search for transition from a psychology grounded in one-way dialectical materialism to a psychology based upon two-way dialectical materialism was marked by intellectual struggle to maintain a balance between good science and acceptable politics. The writings and research of K.N. Kornilov, head of the prestigious Moscow Institute of Psychology during the 1920s, demonstrate the difficulty of the transition.

In formulating his school of reactology, Kornilov deliberately endeavored to make direct contact with Marxist doctrine. He asserted that while nonreflexive thought and movement were necessary, a true psychology must include the even prior consequences that follow from the production of labor. He pulled together his position in a paper addressed especially to American psychologists. He stated:

Marxian psychology, along with the biological elements, attaches still greater importance to social agencies and to their influence on man's behavior, ... from the Marxian standpoint man became a man, the social animal with the most highly developed psychophysiological system, with the gift of speech and thought, only because he began during the process of adaptation to his environment *to prepare* tools for production. Labor and the processes of labor—these are the sources from which sprang the biological changes in the structure of the human organism. Thus labor turned man into a social animal connected with others by complex ties.

Articulate speech grew out of these social relations of labor, and together with this its subjective expression, thinking in words, an indispensible medium for any ideological work.

Thus, everything that is human, everything that distinguishes man from the beasts, is, historically speaking, only the product of labor and, in this way, of social relations.[7]

In his research, Kornilov tried to show how the Marxist conception of the role of labor could be examined in the laboratory. His underlying assumption was that "the product of physical and mental energy is a constant."[8] A moment's reflection upon this assumption forces us to a grinding halt. What can his equation possibly mean? Even though most would agree that the mental "energy" involved in writing creatively with a pencil is at least as great as the energy expended in pushing the pencil, is there indeed an inverse relationship between the two, as implied by the equation? If so, how is mental "energy" to be specified?

Many years later. A.R. Luria provided some insight into Kornilov's reasoning and approach:

He [Kornilov] investigated a series of reactions graded in complexity from simple motor reflexes to associative speech responses. By measuring the latent period and amplitude of the motor response, Kornilov attempted to determine those energy losses which characterize the transition to more complex reactive processes. . . . Although the attempt to measure the energy lost in associative processes was based on a clearly false, mechanistic premise, it had a great effect upon the development of a natural-science approach to the study of certain aspects of human behavior.[9]

For example, Kornilov attributed the fact that the reaction time to a complex association is greater relative to the reaction time of a simple motor reflex, to the greater mental energy expended in the former.

Kornilov's theorizing and procedure for inferring the relative strengths of physical and mental energy (qua *energy*) are no longer taken seriously by psychologists. However, the techniques he developed for recording and measuring simple-to-complex associative processes (changes in reaction time, response topography, and speech patterns) have had lasting influence. At least as important is his continuing effect upon the philosophy of Soviet psychology. His emphasis upon the bio-social significance of "processes of labor" is still accepted as dictum in current writings. For example, Lomov (USSR Academy of Sciences) has declared

Soviet psychology believes that the differences between animals and people are primarily qualitative and are determined by a special characteristic of human beings: The main determinants of human life, and of human mind, are work and communication. Abstract thinking, imagination, creativity, indeed human consciousness itself, are products of the development of the human being engaged in the process of work; they are determined by social life, by the structure of society.[10]

While Kornilov was trying to adapt psychology to the Marxist requirements, Pavlov—who was not a party member—was unintentionally and gracefully accomplishing the task.

Pavlov was not a newcomer to the scientific scene. He started his research well before the revolution, and was permitted to go on with it during the revolution. However, it was not until the meeting of the Soviet Academies of Sciences and Medical Sciences held in 1950 that it was officially decided that Pavlov's research on higher nervous activity satisfied the physiological and psychological requirements of two-way dialectical materialism. In order to understand why his work (which led to the Nobel prize in medicine, 1904) was eventually found to be in accord with communist doctrine, we need briefly to review his discovery of conditioning, the laboratory paradigm he used to examine it, and his own interpretation of conditioning's role in human behavior.

Pavlov's main interest as a physiologist was in the digestive system. He had the genius to recognize the experimental utility of the commonplace observation that hungry dogs salivate upon the appearance of their handlers or other external stimuli signaling the forthcoming arrival of food. He was quick to realize that he could examine in the laboratory the transition from a subcortical event (reflexive salivation to food-in-the-mouth), to a cortical event (thus, "*higher* nervous activity," or acquired anticipatory salivation to external signals). Thereby, he could accomplish what Sechenov failed to achieve; namely, the description of psychical activity in a justifiably physiological language.

Simultaneously, and without political motivation, Pavlov made apparent that his conditioning theory and techniques were amenable to the requirements of two-way dialectical materialism, and he did so with perspicacity. He wrote:

It is quite clear that the activity of even such apparently insignificant organs as the salivary glands penetrates unconsciously into our everyday psychical conditions *through sensations, desires, and thoughts which in turn exert an influence on the work of the glands themselves.* We see no reason why the same should not apply to the other organs of the body. It is, indeed, by means of such impressions that the usual physiological processes of our bodies are guided.[11]

At about the same time that Pavlov reported his discovery of salivary conditioning, C.S. Sherrington independently discovered heart-rate conditioning. Sherrington, another Nobel prize winner in medicine (1932), was doing research on vasomotor reflexes, and was also using dogs as subjects. His procedure involved passing electrical currents through selected nerves. Before energizing his leads, he would carefully check and calibrate his source of voltage, a small transformer called an inductorium.

Sherrington noted that following each such shock-free check, his recordings indicated a depression in heart rate of his subject. He finally realized that his dogs were responding to a signal of impending shock, the audible hum which often accompanies the passage of current through the wires of a transformer. Even though the animals were not actually shocked during the calibration of the inductorium, they responded because of their anticipation of the shock. Sherrington was fully cognizant of the importance of this phenomenon. He published his findings in the *Proceedings of the Royal Society* (1902), under the title "Experiments on the Value of Vascular and Visceral Factors in the Genesis of Emotion." Unlike Pavlov, he then dropped his interest in conditioning. However, "His prototype, more than Pavlov's perhaps, catches the imagination today. After all, one is not so much concerned in his everyday life, with whether or not his mouth waters. He is more concerned with trauma and preparation for trauma. Quite clearly, Sherrington's work falls into this pattern." [12]

Pavlov's and Sherrington's cases of conditioning are dissimilar in that one involves an appetitive situation, and the other an aversive. Nonetheless, a single paradigm is sufficient to describe both. There are two steps to the procedure (the symbol "→" means "is followed by"):

Step. 1. *Pairing of stimuli*
conditioned stimulus → unconditioned stimulus → unconditioned response
Step 2. *Emergence of conditioned response*
CS → CR → US → UR

At this point, a cautionary note is in order: The CS does not functionally replace the US, as is implied by the "stimulus substitution" theory. If the CS served only to substitute for the US, then it follows logically that the response to the CS (the CR) would be the same as the response to the US (the UR), which is not the case. Indeed, Pavlov himself commented that: "A further essential difference between the old |inborn| and the new reflexes is that the former are constant and unconditioned, while the latter are subject to fluctuation, and dependent upon many conditions. They, therefore, deserve the name 'conditioned' [originally, conditional]."[13]

Elsewhere, Pavlov commented that the CS *becomes a surrogate* for the US, and in that sense only is a substitute. However, the substitution is of a "stands for" or designative type, not one of equivalency; otherwise, the CR and UR indeed would be identical. Jenkins and Moore (1973) provided this enlightening quotation from Pavlov:

The first reaction elicited by the established conditioned stimulus usually consists in a movement towards the stimulus, i.e., the animal turns to the place where the [conditioned] stimulus is to be found [not necessarily where the US is to be delivered]. If the stimulus is within reach, the animal even tries to come in touch with it, namely, by means of its mouth. Thus if the conditioned stimulus is the switching on of a lamp, the dog licks the lamp; if the conditioned stimulus is a sound, the dog will even snap in the air (in the case of very heightened food excitability). In this way the conditioned stimulus actually stands for the animal in place of food.[14]

As put by R.S. Woodworth and M.R. Sheehan:

The "stimulus substitution" theory suggests, incorrectly, that the CS—when conditioning has taken place—produces the actual reflex connected with the US. . . . Closely related to this point is the error in thinking that the CR is the same as the natural reflex. . . . The CR is a *preparatory* response made in advance to the signal of food—a getting ready for the receiving of the food, while the reflex is a *consummatory* response to the food itself. So too with defensive and other kinds of reflex behavior.[15]

In point of fact, even the chemical constituents of CR saliva and of UR saliva are different. Similarly, the cardiac CR to a signal indicating that shock is forthcoming, is either a depression or an acceleration depending upon the procedures used, even though the UR to shock is always an acceleration.[16]

All told, Pavlov's main contribution to psychology was to show how physiological terminology and technique could be used to describe and to study modifications in glandular function. He successfully integrated aspects of associationism (the pairing of stimuli), reflexology (the importance of inborne reflexes), and of functionalism (the preparatory qualities of the CR). He pointed the way to what is now known in the Soviet as psychophysiology, a discipline that includes most of what is called experimental psychology in the United States and elsewhere.

Other behavioral scientists of the revolutionary period were interested in the consequences of an organism's *interaction* with the environment, and not solely in internal, glandular phenomena. V.M. Bekhterev studied skeletal muscle conditioning in an aversive situation, using human subjects. He appears to have been the first to examine motor avoidance behavior. Here the US was shock-to-the-finger, and the UR was finger withdrawal. The two steps in his paradigm are as follows (the symbol "$\nrightarrow$" means "is not followed by"):

Step 1. Pairing of stimuli

CS $\longrightarrow$ US $\longrightarrow$ UR
(light)   (shock)   (finger withdrawal)

Step 2. Emergence of conditioned response

CS $\longrightarrow$ CR $\xrightarrow{\quad\nrightarrow\quad}$ US $\nrightarrow$ UR
(light)   (finger withdrawal)   (shock)   (finger withdrawal)

Bekhterev's research is particularly important, since the ability to use external signals in order to avoid dangerous environmental situations is vital to survival. The finger-withdrawal response in Step 1 is reflexive; it is not in Step 2.

J. Konorski and S. Miller initiated the use of a combination of aversive and appetitive control in motor conditioning. Their paradigm is especially interesting in that the procedure involves motor behavior that is first induced reflexively for a few trials, through mildly aversive stimulation. Each such trial is then followed by food reinforcement. They used dogs as subjects.

Step 1. Pairing of stimuli

CS $\longrightarrow$ US $\longrightarrow$ UR $\longrightarrow$ US $\longrightarrow$ UR
(placement in cage) (mild shock to leg) (leg flexion) (food) (eating)

Soon conditioned (or non-reflexive) leg flexion occurs when the dog is placed in the cage. The shock is no longer required to elicit the behavior.

Step 2. Emergence of conditioned response

CS ⟶ CR ⟶ US ⟶ UR

(placement in cage)   (leg flexion)   (food)   (eating)

This type of "push-pull" conditioning is useful when the pure or applied scientist wishes to select a motor response for positive reinforcement, but finds that the response has a low emission rate. Skinner later devised means whereby a selected sample of motor behavior occurred with sufficient frequency (the bar-pressing, "free operant") and could be reinforced with food directly, without having first to be elicited reflexively.[17]

Postrevolutionary Times

We will now examine specific examples illustrating how and why the research of postrevolutionary psychophysiologists satisfied the doctrine of two-way dialectical materialism. We will see what they actually did in the laboratory to substantiate Pavlov's claim "that the activity of even such apparently insignificant organs as the salivary glands penetrates unconsciously into our everyday psychical conditions through sensations, desires and thoughts which in turn exert an influence on the work of the glands themselves."

G. Razran described the following experiment, originally reported by Soviet scientists.[18] A 13-year-old boy was admitted to a surgical ward for an operation involving the salivary glands. Permission was received for the patient to participate as a subject in conditioning research. In one experiment, he was conditioned to secrete saliva to the numerical thought of "10," and to inhibit secretion to "8." Any arithmetic procedure yielding "10" (e.g., $83 - 73$, or $1000 \div 100$) was positively reinforced; any procedure yielding "8" was negatively reinforced. The dramatic results of the experiment are depicted in table 5.1. The columns labeled "Arithmetical Operations Tested," and "Salivary Drops in 30 Sec." tell the story.

Table 5.1 Salivation of 13-year-old boy to different arithmetical operations after he had been conditioned positively to "10" and negatively to "8." (From Razran 1961)

Trial No.	Time of Experimentation		Arithmetical Operations Tested	Test No.	Salivary Drops in 30 Sec.
	Date	Exact Time			
1	8/12/52	11:10'00"	83 − 73	1	15
2		11:14'00"	5 + 5	1	16
3		11:18'30"	20 − 12	1	2
4		11:20'30"	1000 ÷ 100	1	18
5		11:24'30"	5 × 2	1	19
6		11:28'00"	56 ÷ 7	1	2
7		11:32'00"	24 − 14	1	19
8	8/14/52	13:15'00"	19 − 9	1	7
9		13:19'00"	8 + 2	1	19
10		13:22'30"	48 ÷ 6	1	3
11		13:23'30"	4 × 2	1	2
12		13:24'00"	80 ÷ 8	1	17
13		13:27'30"	112 − 102	1	11
14		13:29'30"	4 + 4	1	3
15		13:31'30"	470 ÷ 47	1	11
16	8/14/52	13:33'00"	99 − 91	1	3
17		13:35'00"	80 ÷ 8	2	21
18		13:38'00"	88 ÷ 11	1	3
19		13:40'30"	35 − 25	1	25

In another experiment, the same subject was conditioned to salivate to the word *khorosho* (meaning "good" or "well"), and to inhibit secretion to *plokho* (meaning "poorly," "badly," "bad"). Generalization to sentences or phrases having the good or bad connotations was then tested. Table 5.2 shows how effectively the "insignificant salivary glands" reflect semantic generalization, and incidentally are quite revealing of the kinds of values inculcated by Soviet society.

A major challenge for Soviet scientists was to elucidate upon what Lomov has referred to as the "qualitative" difference between animals and people (see p. 85). One strategy is to examine the interaction between exteroceptive (mainly visual) and kinesthetic governance of motor behavior, an inquiry which began with Sechenov's reflexology, continued through Kornilov's reac-

Table 5.2 Salivation of 13-year-old boy to various words and phrases after he had been conditioned positively to the word *khorosho* |well, good| and negatively to the word *plokha* |poorly, badly, bad|. (From Razran 1961)

| Trial No. | Time of Experimentation | | Words or Phrases Tested | Test No. | Salivary Drops in 30 Sec. |
	Date	Exact Time			
1	6/26/52	11:20'00"	*khorosho*	47	9
2		11:25'15"	*Uchenik prekrasno zani-mayet-sya* |The pupil studies excellently.|	1	14
3		11:29'15"	*Deti igrayut khorosho* |The children are playing well.|	1	19
4		11:31'15"	*plokho*	11	2
5		11:32'45"	*khorosho*	48	15
6		11:37'00"	*Sovet-skaya Armiya pobedila* |The Soviet Army was victorious.|	1	23
7		11:42'00"	*Uchenik nagrubil ychitel'nitse* |The pupil was fresh to the teacher.|	1	0
8		11:45'15'	*khorosho*	49	18
9		11:49'45"	*Pioner pomogayet tovarishchu* |The pioneer helps his comrade.|	1	23
10	7/31/52	10:10'00"	*khorosho*	50	18
11		10:14'00"	*plokho*	12	1
12		10:17'00"	*khorosho*	50	16
13		10:21'00"	*Leningrad—zamechatel'ny gorod* |Leningrad is a wonderful city.|	1	15
14		10:24'30"	*Shkol'nik ne sdal ekzamen* |The pupil failed to take the examination.|	1	2
15		10:26'00"	*khorosho*	52	15

tology, and has been sustained in several modes of conditioning. The issue of which type of cue is more salient on a developmental basis to which type of species, is important because it may explain the more adaptable behavior of the human being. Investigators at the Leningrad laboratory found that for the ape, kinesthetic cues dominate visual cues, and do so even for the mature adult. Their conclusion rests mainly upon experiments done with a single chimpanzee, Rafael.[19] (More will be said about the Russian research with primates when we consider gestalt psychology, since they interpreted their experiments as constituting a refutation of Kohler's work.) A.V. Zaporozhets reported a similar tendency for kinesthetic dominance in human beings, but only up to about 4.5 years of age (see figure 5.1).[20] From that point on, human beings rely much more upon visual stimuli, especially those involved in initial familiarization with (i.e., orientation toward) objects in the environment. Eventually, even imitation-learning can occur by means of vision alone. Taken together, the propensities for visual orientation and imitation learning constitute a crucial step forward in behavioral adaptation and biological evolution. Zaporozhets also indicated that visual-motor skills can gradually become so routine as to require little concurrent feedback during their execution. Such is the case because human beings can learn rapidly (even through verbal instructions) to utilize initiating cues that trigger off a whole train of motor behavior. In today's terms, we call such behavior "motor programs," actions that reveal the

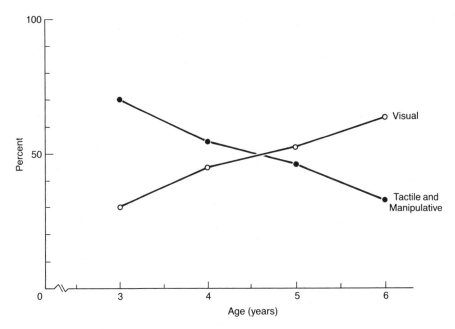

Figure 5.1 Orientative activity of preschool children upon initial familiarization with new objects, expressed as a percentage. (Data shown are reduced from Zaporozhets 1960, table 3)

functional organization of entire segments of limb or body movements.

A.R. Luria explored further the "qualitative" distinctions of man by examining the developmental interactions between the human being's observation of the environment and the emergence of language and thought.[21] He discovered that for children learning how to talk, the *initial* form of paired-associative speech is as follows: If the stimulus-word was an object (a noun, such as "dog"), then the response-word consisted of an action (a verb, such as "bark"). This stage was followed by object-object associations (e.g., "dog"-"cat"). The latter associations are mainly acquired in school. The importance of this finding exists in the fact that—right from the start—the developing human organism learns how to talk in a manner that reflects an active interrelation between him and the environment. The *particular* environment, in turn, influences the kinds of language and thought that ensue, a psychological fact of enormous social-political significance.

From these initial, primitive, paired-word associations, the child begins to attach meaning (or semantic content) to words. At first, these meanings are bound to the physical attributes of the objects or actions from which they stem. Thus, the dog-cat association might lead to the limited, *designative* concept of "four-legs" or "furry." Eventually, the child generalizes to broader concepts. Thus, increasing exposure to the dog-cat type of association, but with other creatures, leads eventually to the more sophisticated concept, "animal." The concept "animal" is semantically distinguished from "non-animal" increasingly through numerous, finer, more subtle discriminations, perhaps abetted by a course in biology. The process continues evolving in adolescence, and perhaps even beyond.

Luria held that verbal behavior and thought (including consciousness) could not be equated with each other. Each has its own set of rules. It is a materialistic error to equate thought with internal verbal behavior, or implicit speech. Luria did for *speech* and thought what Kulpe did for *visual images* and thought. Even as Kulpe demonstrated that thought could take place without visual images, so Luria and his associates demonstrated that thought can occur without implicit speech, *or* visual images, *or* grammatical rules, *or* logical rules—although the *development* of thought is never completely independent of them.

Parenthetically it may be remarked, in the context of our noting relations between verbal and other behavior, that human adults can make use of *verbal* information given to indicate that an aversive US will no longer follow a CS affecting *autonomic* responses. The information hastens, but does not entirely produce, the extinction of an autonomic CR (see figure 5.2). If the same information is combined with an instructed, *motor-avoidance* response, however, then extinction takes place almost immediately.[22] The implications for psychotherapy, particularly behavior modification, are considered later in the book.

Finally, N.A. Bernshtein has suggested that the ideas of cybernetics can be used to illuminate the "qualitatively" different behavior of human beings.[23] Among other matters, he considered how the neuroanatomical properties of physiological systems allow the processing of time-derivative information, thereby

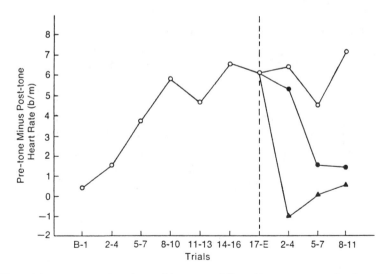

Figure 5.2 Acquisition of conditioned heart rate, followed by extinction under three different procedures: noninstructed, instructed, and instructed-avoidance. (From Notterman, Schoenfeld, and Bersh 1952)

permitting the emergence of anticipatory responses. Although he wrote as a physiologist and cybernetician, his approach is compatible with the behavioral analysis and data contained in chapter 3. One of his statements serves to pull together the contributions of the other Soviet scientists, briefly described in the preceding pages: "The natural materialists [one-way] failed to recognize that a reflex is not an element of an action, but rather an elementary action, because they underestimated the decisive fact of the wholeness and systematic nature of an organism and its function."[24] As we saw earlier in the chapter, John Dewey expressed the same sentiment.

Summary Comment

Many of us conclude our studies in psychology with a conception of classical conditioning that is a caricature of its true nature. Oddly, we Americans tend to view classical conditioning within the constraints of one-way dialectical materialism. We perceive Pavlovian conditioning to be some sort of rigid, elementalistic, switchlike approach to psychological inquiry. It is not. We tend to be unfamiliar with the rich contributions of the Soviet scientists in fields that *we* separate into cognitive psychology, neuropsychology, psycholinguistics, and so on. The Russian investigators consider—for historical and political reasons—such research to be part and parcel of a two-way dialectical-materialist approach to "psychophysiology." We overreact to the narrowness conjured up by this word. Politics aside, there is little difference between Russian psychophysiology and American general experimental psychology.

6 American Behaviorism: Watsonian and Skinnerian Versions

T he first objective of this chapter is to look carefully at behaviorism's origins in J.B. Watson's declarative writings, and at behaviorism's extensions in B.F. Skinner's research-oriented works. The second objective is to place Skinnerian behaviorism in the broader context of the other forms of psychological inquiry thus far examined.

Initial Reception of Watson's and Skinner's Versions of Behaviorism

At about the time that Titchener and Kulpe were raising doubts about structuralism, the *Psychological Review* published Watson's article, "Psychology as the Behaviorist Views It.".[1] This paper rapidly became known as his "manifesto." Watson then wrote a book to bring his message to the layman. The reviews of this book verged on the ecstatic: "Some of the excitement generated by Watson's ideas can be appreciated from the newspaper reviews of *Behaviorism*. The *New York Times* said dramatically, 'It marks an epoch in the intellectual history of man' (August 2, 1925); the *New York Herald Tribune* commented, 'Perhaps this is the most important book ever written. One stands for an instant blinded with a great hope.'"[2]

Twenty-five years after Watson's manifesto, B.F. Skinner published his detailed research volume, *The Behavior of Organisms: An Experimental Analysis* (1938). By 1966, it had gone through seven printings. Because of his creative work in operant conditioning, and because of his many subsequent extrapolative writings regarding human behavior, Skinner became the most widely known of twentieth-century American psychologists. A 1975 survey found that he was correctly identified by 82 percent of a college student sample, heading a list of the top twenty American scientists of *all* fields.[3] Of course, recognition does not necessarily imply approval. Visibility is as often due to opposition as it is to concurrence. But that is beside the main point: behaviorism has profoundly influenced psychological inquiry. We shall inspect the Watsonian and Skinnerian varieties separately, in an effort to identify and to evaluate the essence of the two approaches.

Watsonian Behaviorism

We begin by briefly citing the salient portions of Watson's often misconstrued manifesto, commenting on each in turn. Thereby, we will more accurately convey and assess the raison d'etre of early behaviorism.

What Watson in Fact Said About Psychology

1. "I feel that *behaviorism* is the only consistent and logical functionalism."[4] In light of this statement, it appears that Watson intended to correct or to extend functionalism, not to abandon it.

2. "The psychology which I should attempt to build up would take as a starting point, first, the observable fact that organisms, man and animal alike, do adjust themselves to their environment by means of heredity and habit equipments." Watson indicated that functionalism's primary concern—the phenomenon of adaptation—was open to scientific examination, and

therefore should be retained in a behavioristic approach to psychology.

3. "I believe we can write a psychology . . . and . . . never use the term consciousness, mental states, mind, content, introspectively verifiable, imagery, and the like." Watson asserted that psychology should not be concerned with mental phenomena. He departed from functionalism in this important respect, for reasons made apparent in the next quotation.

4. "The consideration of the mind-body problems affects neither the type of problem selected nor the formulation of the solution of that problem." He was neither a parallelist nor an interactionist. The implication is that behaviorists are not dualists of any sort. We shall shortly return to this assertion.

5. "The behaviorist, in his efforts to get a unitary scheme of animal response, recognizes no dividing line between man and brute." He argued, in Darwinian fashion, for a comparative psychology. This is consistent with functionalist doctrine.

The following is not a direct quotation from Watson, but from Woodworth and Sheehan, summarizing Watson's viewpoint. "There is no mystery in the relation of body and behavior. Psychologists have introduced unnecessary mystery by replacing the mind or soul by the inaccessible brain. Behaviorism must not make a fetish of the brain but must keep its eyes fixed on the peripheral organs, the sense organs, muscles and glands."[5] Watson criticized the American functionalist emphasis on the brain, as it had turned a broadly conceived physiological psychology into a narrower "brain psychology." He wanted behaviorism to avoid that mistake.

What Watson Did Not Say About Psychology

1. By emphasizing "the observable fact" that organisms adjust to the environment, Watson did *not* mean to restrict the psychologist's field of observation to extra-ectodermic events: i.e., to the exclusive study of gross movement or of limb action. Indeed, he used the term "implicit behavior" to describe responses that were not directly observable with the naked eye. Im-

plicit behavior such as nerve impulses and visceral, glandular, and proprioceptive responses were, given proper instrumentation, potentially as accessible to observation as overt behavior. By "fact," then, he implied any event that lent itself to counting or measuring operations, and to independent verification of these operations by other observers.

2. Watson did not deny the *presence* of consciousness. He did deny that consciousness could be reliably introspected by even a trained subject, and maintained that appeals to consciousness as a source of behavior had no scientifically valid, explanatory value.

3. Watson insisted that psychology was a field separate from physiology, and that attempts to *reduce* the former to the latter were futile. However, Watson did not reject the importance of a general physiological psychology, or of relating the physiological and the psychological to each other. For instance, he did not dissociate behaviorism from psychophysiology's Pavlovian conditioning. In fact, Watson's S-R model of behavior was not only quite compatible with Pavlov's, but was also influenced by it.

Transition from Watsonian to Skinnerian Behaviorism

Disclaimers notwithstanding, early behaviorism gradually drifted toward an exclusive concern with directly "observable facts" of a particular type; namely, movement responses. The reason for this development was probably the ease of instrumentation and the convenience of experimentation inherent in such research.

Despite Watson's lack of concern with mind-body dualism, the preoccupation with movements led to an investigatory emphasis upon limb actions, thus effectively restoring the very dichotomy so earnestly condemned. Moreover, not only was the mind excluded, but also the viscera, glands, and muscles. "Limb-action," as examined through Skinner's bar-pressing procedure, became the primary technical concern of behaviorists.

Skinnerian Behaviorism

As with Watson, Skinner's conception of the proper subject matter of psychology in general, and of behaviorism in particular, requires careful scrutiny. In part, this need exists because of the tendency to distort, favorably or unfavorably, the viewpoint of any prominent figure to render it consistent with one's own outlook. However, there are two other reasons for the prevalence of mistaken notions concerning Skinnerian behaviorism. First, his research reports demand the reader's most careful attention, and the writing style is not particularly accommodating. This is particularly troublesome in his landmark volume, *Behavior of Organisms*. Second, his position on various issues appears to be ambiguous, and even to have changed with the years. For some, this is distressing; for others, it is a sign of Skinner's dynamic genius. We shall consider three of these apparent ambiguities, using his own words to illustrate each instance. They lend themselves to consideration as "definitions of behavior and its properties."

Definitions of Behavior and Its Properties
1. On *behavior, movement, and effect*. "By behavior, then, I mean simply the *movement of an organism or of its parts* in a frame of reference provided by the organism itself or by various external objects or fields of force. It is convenient to speak of this as the action of the organism upon the outside world, *and it is often desirable to deal with an effect rather than with the movement itself.*"[6]

Watson originally emphasized the description of observable facts, based upon the premise that implicit behavior was potentially observable. He did not intend to restrict psychology to an examination of an organism's movements. Skinner declared that he *was* interested exclusively in the movement of the organism or of its parts, since it was only through action that the organism could affect the environment. Perhaps he did so because it was crucial to his distinction between two types of conditioning, respondent and operant (or classical and instrumental). In the respondent case, appearance of the US—e.g., food for the Pavlovian dog—is not contingent upon any prior response (autonomic or motor) of the organism. The food arrives whether or not the dog salivates. In the operant case, appearance of the US (again, assume food), awaits some specific action (or operation) by the organism, one which has a particular effect upon the environment. Operant conditioning involves response-contingent reinforcement. Two commonly used laboratory responses are bar-pressing (rats), or key-pecking (pigeons). Any device used for response-contingent reinforcement is termed a "manipulandum."

Returning to the quotation, note the important qualification in the last sentence; namely that it is frequently preferable to deal with the *effect* of the action (or movement), rather than with the action itself. With the years, the "often desirable" became the general rule. The difference between examining an action per se, and determining the effect of the action, translates itself into the difference between describing changes in the nature or contents of an action, and counting how often the action—regardless of its internal fluctuations—occurs in time. We shall have more to say about the importance of this difference when we look more closely at the bar-pressing technique.

2. On *behavior and purpose.* "In English . . . we say that an organism . . . *has a purpose, tries,* and *succeeds* or *fails* . . . these terms must be avoided in a scientific description of behavior."[7]

Skinner went on to argue that even if these vernacular expressions could be defined operationally, as was attempted by the early behaviorists, it would be to no avail. The expressions, no matter how carefully defined, rest upon flawed cultural assumptions concerning the actual sources of behavior. For example, behavior originates and is sustained by reinforcement contingencies, not by inherently "good" or "evil" motives. His position is convincingly stated. But in the Preface to the seventh printing of *Behavior of Organisms*, the following clause appears: "operant behavior is the field of purpose."[8] Even the earnest reader is initially puzzled by the apparent inconsistency. Of course, the words are intended to convey the idea that a scientific analysis of operant behavior precludes the necessity for dealing with the layman's conceptual schema of "purpose."

   3. On *behavior and biology*.

The use of the nervous system as a fictional explanation of behavior was a common practice even before Descartes, and it is now much more widely used than is generally realized. At a popular level a man is said to be capable (a fact about his behavior) because he has brains (a fact about his nervous system). Whether or not such a statement has any meaning for the person who makes it is scarcely important; in either case it exemplifies the practice of explaining an obvious (if unorganized) fact by appeal to something about which little is known. The more sophisticated neurological views generally agree with the popular view in contending that behavior is in itself incomprehensible but may be reduced to law if it can be shown to be controlled by an internal system susceptible to scientific treatment. *Facts about behavior are not treated in their own right, but are regarded as something to be explained or even explained away by the prior facts of the nervous system.* (I am not attempting to discount the importance of a science of neurology but am referring simply to the primitive use of the nervous system as an explanatory principle in avoiding a direct description of behavior).[9]

   The key point here is that a science of behavior should develop its own language, and that "facts about behavior" cannot be (and should not be) reduced to facts about biology. But in a much more recent positional statement, the following appears: "I must begin by saying what I take a science of behavior to be. It is, I assume, part of biology. The organism that behaves is the organism that breathes, digests, conceives, gestates, and so on. As such, the behaving organism will eventually be described and explained by the anatomist and physiologist."[10] Of course, Skinner goes on to say that "eventually" is a long time off, and that a science based upon reinforcement contingencies will nonetheless remain useful, and even guide the physiologist and anatomist in their task of describing and explaining behavior. But the question for us as students of psychology is whether that particular eventual description is the *kind* of description in which the psychologist is (or should be) fundamentally interested.

We have sufficiently examined Watson's and Skinner's definitions of behavior to have placed the writings of both figures in some critical perspective. In good behavioristic fashion, we will now set aside the writings, and examine the laboratory techniques. We shall focus upon Skinner's well-known bar-pressing procedure.

Procedure Followed in Bar-pressing Conditioning

If the reader has not had "hands-on" experience in the animal laboratory, he may have the impression that the conditioning of bar-pressing is a fairly "automatic" procedure. The rat is placed into a Skinner box, and is envisioned as quite routinely beginning to press the bar with its paw and to receive pellets. Such is hardly the case. It is not only bar-pressing that is conditioned, but also prior links in a chain of behavior, very much in the manner of James Mill's mechanical associationism. The following account of what Skinnerians call "chaining," describes the steps involved, when the experimenter aims to condition the rat to press a bar and to do so only in the presence of a light-on signal.

Hunger rhythm: Starting about a week before the actual conditioning session, and continuing throughout the experiment, the rat is placed on a daily fast of 22–23 hours. During the 24th hour, the rat is fed some mash mixed with the pellets of food that will eventually be used as reinforcement. Pellets are mixed with the mash so that the rat will learn to recognize them as food, and get accustomed to eating them. The hour or two between fast and feeding is reserved for the future experimental period, beginning with tray-approach training.

Tray-approach training: The Skinner box has a tray inside, just below and to the side of a horizontal bar (or lever)

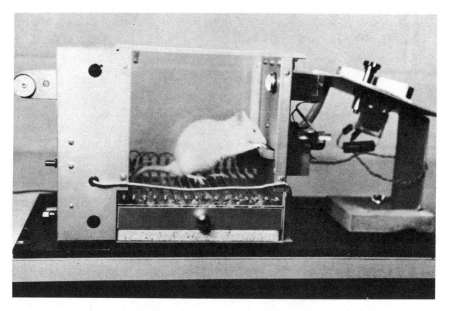

Figure 6.1 Typical Skinner box. (From Notterman 1970)

mounted on a wall, and extending through to the outside of the cage. When the bar is depressed completely, it closes a switch outside the cage, thereby completing a circuit to a pellet-dispenser and to recording devices. Switch closure is accompanied by a click. The experimenter uses this click to train the hungry animal to obtain a pellet in the tray, as soon as the click is produced. He begins by watching carefully until he sees the rat happen to approach the tray. When the rat's nose is near the tray, he quickly depresses the lever from *outside* the box, thereby closing the switch, producing a click, and energizing the pellet dispenser. The goal is to train the rat to approach the tray as soon as the click occurs. Toward this end, the experimenter must also be certain to provide occasions during which the rat's approach to the tray is not preceded by the click-pellet pairing. When tray-approaches not preceded by the click go unreinforced, they extinguish. The lamp inside the box is kept on throughout, because the aim is to have light-on eventually serve as a signal for when to press. Ordinarily, it takes one or two sessions to establish the click-discrimination outlined in the following expression (note that "S^D" is the abbreviation for *discriminative stimulus*, or cue for responding; "S$^\Delta$" (ess-delta), the abbreviation for the *absence of* S^D; "$\rightarrow$" means *is followed by*; "$\nrightarrow$" means *is not followed by*; "R" means *response*):

$$S^D_{(click)} \rightarrow R_{(tray\ approach)} \rightarrow pellet$$

$$S^\Delta_{(no\ click)} \rightarrow R_{(tray\ approach)} \nrightarrow pellet$$

Bar-pressing training: With the lamp still on, the experimenter waits until the animal presses the bar all the way down with one of its forepaws. To accomplish this action, the rat must exert sufficient force to overcome the elastic resistance of a spring within the switch. The click occurs as soon as the contact points have been closed. Ideally, the animal then releases the bar, drops to the tray, and obtains its pellet. The pellet is not delivered until the bar is released, thus precluding the development of what is called "holding" behavior. If the animal presses the bar with insufficient force to close the switch, there is no click, a response is not registered, and a pellet is not received.

Bar-pressing conditioning is underway, as assessed by an increase in rate of responding. The following expressions apply: (The symbol

$$R_{(\text{"bar–pressing"})}$$

means that the bar has not been fully displaced; i.e., it has been pressed with insufficient force to close the switch.)

$$R_{(bar-pressing)} \rightarrow S^D_{click} \rightarrow R_{(t.a.)} \rightarrow pellet$$

$$R_{(\text{"bar–pressing"})} \rightarrow S^\Delta_{(no\ click)} \rightarrow R_{(t.a.)} \nrightarrow pellet$$

"Light-on" discrimination training: The experimenter specifies intervals for the lamp in the box to be on and off. These intervals (ranging from several seconds to a couple of minutes) are of quasi-random duration, and are alternated within any single session. The idea is to provide circumstances such that the animal is reinforced only when the light is on, and then only when

it presses hard enough to close the switch. The following expressions summarize the situation:

Light-on

$$S^D_{(light-on)} \rightarrow R_{(b-p)} \rightarrow S^D_{(click)} \rightarrow R_{(t.a.)} \rightarrow (pellet)$$

$$S^D_{(light-on)} \rightarrow R_{("b-p")} \rightarrow S^\Delta_{(no\ click)} \rightarrow R_{(t.a.)} \nrightarrow (pellet)$$

Light-off

$$S^\Delta_{(light-off)} \rightarrow R_{(b-p)} \rightarrow S^D_{(click)} \rightarrow R_{(t.a.)} \nrightarrow (pellet)$$

$$S^\Delta_{(light-off)} \rightarrow R_{("b-p")} \rightarrow S^\Delta_{(no\ click)} \rightarrow R_{(t.a.)} \nrightarrow (pellet)$$

The description so far implies that the animal depends upon presentation of the light to learn when to press, and upon obtaining the click to learn how hard to press. External governance of behavior is emphasized in both the "when" and the "how." The latter requires further elaboration. Apart from the external click, laboratory evidence indicates that, at least initially, the rat also depends upon concurrent, response-produced stimuli (proprioceptive feedback from the response itself) in learning to discriminate the required level of force.[11] Additional findings, fathered with human subjects, indicate that once an action is learned, the need diminishes to discriminate concurrently produced, proprioceptive feedback *during* an action. These findings describe how motor programs become established and unfold.[12]

A Closer Look at Form and Content of Response

In any science, the techniques that are predominantly in use tend to determine the kinds of questions asked. Unless we are careful to keep alert to the fundamental assumptions upon which the methodology rests, the field of inquiry soon becomes constrained to the sort of questions that are amenable mainly to the techniques employed. By attending principally to the rate of bar-pressing response (or rate of effects, or switch-closures), and by largely disregarding the properties of the action per se, such variations as may occur in the character of the action itself inadvertently come to be regarded as essentially random, noninformative, or trivial. In other words, the action becomes no more than its effect, as represented by the closing of a switch.

In this section, we briefly review three relevant studies. They demonstrate that both the structure (e.g., form) and the contents (e.g., force) of individual actions are systematically related to the variables typically used in operant conditioning, such as drive and reinforcement contingency. Ordinarily the influence of these independent variables is assessed through changes in the *rate* of bar-pressing or key-pecking, rather than through changes in the *character* of individual actions. This is not to suggest that the latter avenue of approach is "better" than the former, but only to say that both are necessary to a full conceptualization and analysis of operant conditioning.

Drive and Form of Key-pecking Response

H.M. Jenkins and B.R. Moore pursued a discovery originally made by Ferster and Skinner (1957), who "found that the rate of response in thirsty pigeons receiving water as the reinforcer was lower than for hungry pigeons receiving grain as the reinforcer."[13] Jenkins and Moore believed that the lower response rate with water than with grain originated from a difference in response-form, as first reported by B.R. Wolin. Wolin had used independent observers to watch how pigeons pecked at targets (discs in a panel of the cage; also called "keys") under the two different drive states.[14] His observers were in sufficient agreement to permit Wolin to conclude

that the form of the pigeon's operant key-contact response depends on the nature of the reinforcer. The food-deprived pigeon receiving grain as the reinforcer was observed to make rapid, short, powerful pecks at the key with the beak open at the moment of contact [using the beak as a "pliers"]. The movement closely resembled that used when pecking grain. On the other hand, the water-deprived pigeon receiving water as the reinforcer pushed its almost closed beak against the key in a slower motion that resembled the drinking response [using the beak as a "straw"].[15]

However, the evidence of anticipatory differences in forms of key-pecking response needed buttressing. The response is made so rapidly (.089 sec. under thirst drive, and .057 under hunger drive) that relying upon visual inspection alone was considered unwise. In a classical conditioning experiment involving the emergence of surrogate-stimulus control, Jenkins and Moore obtained convincing, supportive photographic data.

Each pigeon was deprived of both food and water, and a combined hunger-thirst rhythm was established. The pigeon was then placed in the Skinner box, the front panel of which is illustrated in figure 6.2. When the disc on the left was illuminated with red light for 6 sec. (CS), it signalled the impending availability of water (US). When the disc on the right was lit-up with white stripes for 6 sec. (CS), it signalled the ensuing accessibility of grain (US). The fact that reinforcement was not contingent upon key-pecking makes this a Pavlovian situation. Depending upon the particular CS-US pairing to which the pigeon was randomly exposed, the respective UR was either approach to the water receptacle and drinking, or approach to the food hopper and eating. This Pavlovian procedure is known as "autoshaping," as the subjects are left entirely on their own once they are placed in the box. Proper controls are used to insure that whatever CR's emerge do not result from "superstitious" behavior; i.e., to responses inadvertently reinforced by the experimenter.

We already know from chapter 5 that the stimulus substitution theory would predict the acquisition of two CR's, each appropriate to the respective CS→US→UR sequences. Specifically, the red disc should elicit approach to the water cup (CR), and the white-striped disc should elicit approach to the food hopper (CR). What actually happens is that the pigeons peck at whichever *key* becomes lit, instead of going either to the cup or to the hopper. The findings are shown in figure 6.3. The investigators interpreted the photographic evidence in such manner as

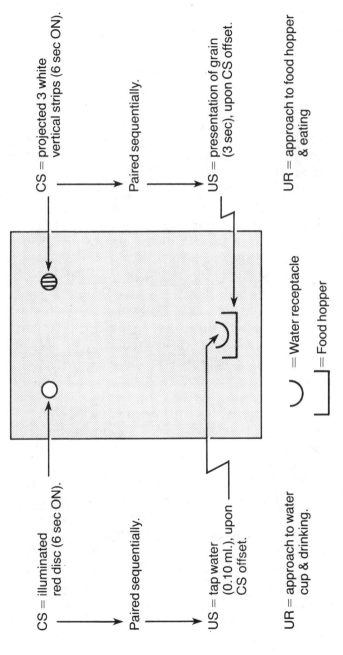

CS = illuminated
red disc (6 sec ON).

Paired sequentially.

US = tap water
(0.10 ml.), upon
CS offset.

UR = approach to water
cup & drinking.

CS = projected 3 white
vertical strips (6 sec ON).

Paired sequentially.

US = presentation of grain
(3 sec), upon CS offset.

UR = approach to food hopper
& eating

⌣ = Water receptacle

⌐⌐ = Food hopper

Figure 6.2 Auto-shaping: Panel used for pigeons in Skinner box. (Jenkins and Moore 1973)

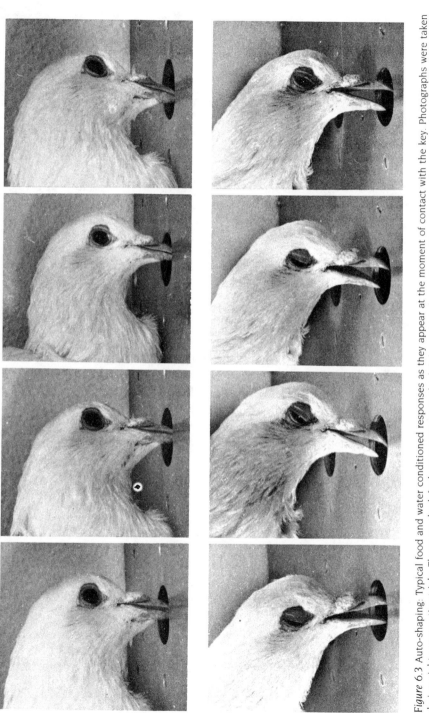

Figure 6.3 Auto-shaping: Typical food and water conditioned responses as they appear at the moment of contact with the key. Photographs were taken during eight consecutive trials. Those on the left show responses to the left key, which was paired with water (see figure 6.2). Those on the right show responses to the right key, which was paired with food. (From Jenkins and Moore 1973), reproduced by permission of the authors)

to dispute the conventional view of the stimulus substitution theory.

The finding that the pigeons peck at the targets even though they do not have to, is intriguing. This discovery of anticipatory (or goal-directed?, or preparatory?) behavior widens the horizons of both operant and classical conditioning. The *difference in form* of the key-pecking response under the two drive states explains Ferster and Skinner's earlier report that operant keypecking for water produces lower rates of responding than does key-pecking for food. We now know *why*, and that knowledge increases our overall understanding of the behavior of organisms.

Reinforcement Contingency and Force of Bar-pressing: Fixed Ratio

In a conventional fixed ratio (FR) schedule of reinforcement, the organism is reinforced after every *n*th response. For example, a rat placed on FR 10 would be reinforced with a pellet after having pressed the bar 10 times in a row. The cycle is then repeated. Typically, FR schedules produce high, fairly constant rates of responding, though the animal pauses briefly after receiving and eating the pellet as if to rest. This kind of schedule is often compared to payment of a laborer on a piece-work basis. It is in the laborer's presumed interest to work as fast as possible, as it is in the animal's.

Notterman and Mintz (1965) used a force-sensitive "bar"—actually the top of a transducer—in a research program concerned with contents of responses. The manipulandum had two other unusual features. First, it was virtually isometric; i.e., its maximal downward displacement was less than a millimeter. The experimenters could thus examine "pure" force emission, without the confounding effects of movement. Second, it was soundless; i.e., there was no click, since there was no switch. Thereby, a premium was placed upon the animal's attending to its own proprioceptive feedback in emitting a response.

A computer measured and recorded the force of the successively emitted responses during FR cycles. For a given contact with the bar to register as a response, it had to peak at at least 2.5 gm of force, and then drop below that level. No higher force was required, either to advance the count in the cycle, or to obtain reinforcement. A major modification from routine FR schedules consisted of the introduction of series of reinforced responses along with the conventional unreinforced responses, during each cycle. Figure 6.4 shows the changes in force that took place for one such FR schedule. The data are from one animal, exposed to 25 cycles per daily session for 15 sessions. Each cycle consisted of 6 reinforced and 12 unreinforced responses. The fact that the changes are quite consistent, even though they were not required of the rat, is noteworthy.

The figure indicates the following: (1) As soon as the animal gets the first pellet in the reinforced portion of the cycle, the level of force drops markedly, and remains low during the remainder of the reinforced series. The reason is that animals tend to exert just enough force, plus a safety margin, to assure reinforcement on most of their responses. (2) As soon as the animal enters the unreinforced portion of the cycle, forces drift upwards, from about 4.5 gm to about 10.5 gm. The regular increase in force is thought to be due to a combination of factors: (1) Emotional energization during a run of unreinforced responding, an effect accompanying extinction. (2) Past history of obtaining reinforcement upon successful completion of a *subsequent* action, if the *prior* action was insufficiently strong to be effectual. (The adage "if at first you don't succeed, try, try again," captures the idea.) (3) Discrimination of increments in response-produced feedback sustains the behavior required to advance the count during a run of unreinforced responding.[16]

Mintz (1962) has shown that the drop in force right after reinforcement, and the gradual increase in force during non-reinforcement, are typical of the conventional FR schedule, one which includes only a single reinforced response.[17]

The major points of the FR studies are that regular changes in force take place during this quite commonly employed

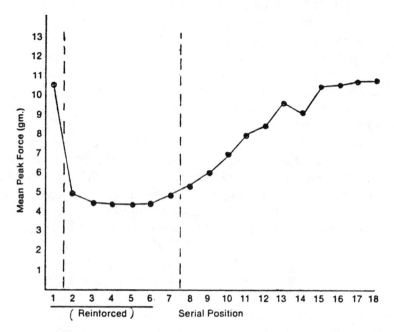

Figure 6.4 Effect upon mean peak force of response, of successively reinforced and non-reinforced cycles of responding. Each point is a mean based upon 375 responses (25 cycles per session x 15 sessions). (After Notterman and Mintz 1965)

type of reinforcement schedule, that these variations occur even though they are not required or induced by the experimenter, that they would go undetected if rate of switch-closures during bar-pressing was used alone as the dependent variable, and that when both rate and force are used as assessments of behavior, each dependent variable helps account for the fluctuations in the other.

Reinforcement Contingency and Force of Bar-pressing: Double Discrimination

In *Behavior of Organisms*, Skinner called attention to the possibility of establishing "double discrimination"—the use of external cues to signal the required emission of a discriminated level of operant response.[18] Some years later, Notterman and Mintz performed an experiment in which they tested Skinner's notion.[19] In publishing their findings, they observed: "This class of behavior has much to teach us, for it deals with a rather commonplace behavioral situation: one in which an organism maintains successive responding, but adjusts each individual response value to that 'required' by the value of a varying exteroceptive cue. This type of behavior is implicit in common forms of closed-loop error detection and correction."[20] The discussion of goal-directed activity and feedback theory in chapter 3 presupposes the existence of just such a capacity for double-discrimination.

We need not go into great detail concerning the research, for figure 6.5 practically tells the story by itself. The figure gives the performance of one rat. "Light-off" in the cage was a signal for pressing between 5 and 10 gm, and "light-on," for pressing within a range or band of 15 and 20 gm. (For four rats, the relationship was as described; for another four, it was reversed to provide a control.) Each of the 41 daily sessions was composed of random presentations of light-on and light-off periods, ranging from 10 to 160 sec. in duration, and accumulating to a total of about 10 minutes for each of the respective signals. The two frequency distributions of forces are clearly separate. (The peak for the higher band falls just below the 15 gm cut-off, and can be accounted for by the principle of least effort, and by the fact that smaller forces are reinforced when the light is off.) Apart from the distributions, the effectiveness of the procedure was indicated by the fact that "the force level of the *first* response following each change in the exteroceptive cue was significantly altered in the appropriate direction."[21] Furthermore, all eight subjects emitted on the average a greater force in the high band than in the low.

While the level of force was required to change with change of external cue, rate of response was left open-ended. It turned out that the group split evenly, with half the subjects responding more often in the higher, and the other half in the lower

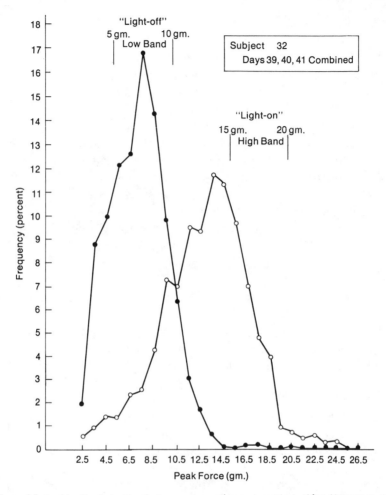

Figure 6.5 Double discrimination (exteroceptive and proprioceptive). (After Notterman and Mintz 1965)

band. Notwithstanding, the animals uniformly obtained more pellets in the low band condition than in the high, as illustrated in figure 6.5.

In summary, the double discrimination research differs from the FR studies in its finding that levels of force are not only internally discriminated, but can be brought under the direct control of external stimuli. The effect of this type of control cannot be demonstrated in any simple fashion by observing only the accompanying rates of bar pressing.[22]

Skinnerian Behaviorism in Perspective

It is time now to call a halt to our examination of the origins and methodologies of behaviorism, and to see how the Skinnerian variety fits into the larger context of psychology's evolution. It is both convenient and instructive to do so in the same sequential order in which other forms of psychological inquiry have been considered so far.

Relation to Cosmology, Spirits, and Animism
Recall that reification means "making a thing out of" a process, and that animism means "the belief that all natural objects and phenomena possess spirits." Spirits are the *things* that account for all that occurs in the world in the rudimentary cosmology of animism.

Today's Western man would hardly agree that he holds animistic views. Yet that is precisely what Skinner has implied through his charge that the modern human being "explains" abstract concepts (such as purpose and free will), by means of homunculi. Instead of treating these abstractions as behaviors originating in reinforcement contingencies, today's person *labels* these behaviors, neglects the *fact* of the labeling, and then attributes causal properties to the labels themselves. It is these labels that then become homunculi—phony, causal agents of behavior. Skinner's most cogent statement of his position appears in *Beyond Freedom and Dignity* (1971).[23] In his piercing review of this work, Noam Chomsky declared:

In support of his belief that science will demonstrate that behavior is entirely a function of antecedent events, Skinner notes that physics advanced only when it "stopped personifying things" and attributing to them "wills, impulses, feelings, purposes," and so on (p. 8). Therefore, he concludes, the science of behavior will progress only when it stops personifying people and avoids reference to "internal states." No doubt physics advanced by rejecting the view that a rock's wish to fall is a factor in its "behavior," because in fact a rock has no such wish. For Skinner's argument to have any force, he must show that people have wills, impulses, feeling, purposes, and the like no more than rocks do. If people do differ from rocks in this respect, then a science of human behavior will have to take account of this fact.[24]

Skinner has not found such criticisms to be devastating. He still maintains: "So long as we cling to the view that a person is an initiating doer, actor, or causer of behavior, we shall probably continue to neglect the conditions which must be changed if we are to solve our problems."[25]

For Skinner, then, a scientifically valid regard for human welfare demands a behavioristic approach, otherwise we fall victim to current forms of primitivistic reification.

Relation to Structuralism

In large measure, the debate between Skinner and Chomsky revolves around the issue of whether mental and affective states, subsumed under the word "internal," can serve as immediate causal agents of behavior. Here we should recall Hilgard's warning that "psychologists and physiologists have to be modest in the face of this problem that has baffled the best philosophical minds for centuries" (chapter 2, p. 35).

Internal states are by definition private matters, and arguments concerning their fundamental character verge on the metaphysical—now, as during the heyday of structuralism. However, the issue of whether the *experience* of thought or free will or purpose can serve as a cause for behavior, and have explanatory value, is important. We shall come back to it.

Relation to Functionalism

The basic character of functionalism is its breadth of view, and particular emphasis upon purposivism. As noted in chapter 3, purposivism has three main attributes: (1) goal-directed activity (James); (2) voluntary change of activity (McDougall); (3) awareness of voluntary action, as expressed by human beings through verbal report (Rosenblueth, Wiener, & Bigelow).

The presence of *awareness* of goal-directed activity, and of voluntary changes in the direction of this activity, is at the heart of the Chomsky-Skinner controversy noted earlier. And to glance ahead to psychoanalysis, we can anticipate still another dispute. Once we accept awareness of changes in voluntary activity as being fundamental to the idea of purpose, it paradoxically leads us to consider the presence of "hidden purpose," or those actions the purposes of which we are unaware. Further, we can easily assign the wrong purpose to an act, in ourselves or in others. In short, we must be cautious in using purpose as an explanation of behavior, and that is exactly Skinner's point. Despite the best of care, the attribution of causal properties to purpose is risky; it is much safer to rely upon reinforcement contingencies as the source of behavior.

We know the retort to this behavioristic viewpoint. Just because the correct assignment of purposes to behavior is challenging, does not mean that we should abandon purposivity as a property of behavior, as seems to be demanded by Skinnerian behaviorism.

Relation to Associationism

Skinnerian behaviorism has roots in associationism's concern with the effects of continguity of events (chapter 4). The earlier discussion of chaining is illustrative.

Through his ideas of chaining, Skinner made a vital contribution to associationism. He developed a methodology whereby each component of a series of stimulus events is dependent upon the organism's prior action. The appropriate cues (discriminative stimuli) do not appear in the chain of behavior, unless preceded by the required response. It is in his methodological emphasis upon a response-dependent contiguity of events leading to reinforcement that Skinner departs from Pavlov. Interestingly, other behaviorists (notably Guthrie) maintained that the *response*-dependent feature of Skinnerian methodology is not important in the development of the organism's associations of links in the chain. It is the presence of contiguity per se between S^D's that is vital, and not the fact that the organism *procures* the next S^D. Experimenters have found evidence both to support and to discredit Guthrie's position. Either way, the researcher's techniques in operant conditioning would remain Skinner's.

Relation to Russian Dialectical-materialist Psychology

The debate between Skinner and Chomsky is reminiscent of the opposing positions taken by the prerevolutionary and postrevolutionary Russians. In both instances, the basic conflict lies in what the antagonists would accept as a causal agent.

For Skinner, causes of behavior cannot be attributed to thought or free will or purpose. These nouns must be reduced to verbs, and the verbs to reinforcement contingencies—to the *consequences* of stimulus-response correlations. In this sense, Skinnerian behaviorism subscribes to Sechenov's analysis of mentation; namely, that autonomous thought, free will, and purpose are illusions—epiphenomena—and cannot be immediate causes of behavior. Indeed, Skinner's most recent definition of behavioral science as being part of biology makes the resemblance with Sechenov even more striking. For Chomsky, causes of behavior *must* be attributed to thought, free will, and purpose. This attribution is crucial, because he works within a philosophical frame of reference, one that requires that he be cognitive, volitional, and purposive. Thus, Chomsky is drawn to a semblance of the position held by two-way dialectical materialism, but for philosophical rather than psychological reasons.

The issue of identifying the "true" determinants of behavior cannot be resolved by disputes between psychologist and philosopher, since each is bound to be "right," according to the rules that he goes by. As students of psychology, we should consider the issue as being between psychologist and psychologist, without becoming so proprietary as to believe we have an exclusive interest in, and understanding of, the matter.

So, as psychologists, let us confront the question: are autonomy of thought, free will, and purposivity incompatible with the principle of determinism, or even with Skinnerian behaviorism? It is possible to answer "No, not necessarily." The behaving organism *does* make choices, and—if human—he can report the experience he has preliminary to the act of choosing. Perhaps what we call free will *is* this experience. Of course, once the choice has been made, it is theoretically possible to search out the antecedent events or reinforcement contingencies that inevitably led to the decision, and thus to disregard the private experience of choosing. However, we generally cannot identify the necessary and sufficient prior circumstances that preceded a choice. Thus, the more proximate *experience* of choosing is reified (or homunculized), and is identified as the cause. In this sense, thought, free will and purpose are indeed epiphenomena.

But we must go one step further, as did the two-way dialectical materialists. We must consider the possibility that our tendency to use nouns and higher abstractions to describe known and unknown reinforcement contingencies is essential to human behavior. Without this tendency, internal thought and communication with others would be virtually impossible. The foregoing is practically a restatement of the two-way dialectical materialist position that "Mentation has its own representative reality . . . and exerts a perceived autonomous influence on an individual's personal and social behavior" (chapter 5, p. 80).

A Finer Statement of the Problem

The foregoing analysis is echoed in biographer Leon Edel's discussion of Henry James's novel, *The Ambassadors*:

In this novel he comes to the question of determinism. He doesn't ask, "What is life?" He accepts life. The question he asks is how much of life

one can live within the restraints of civilization. One may not be tech-
nically a free man; one may be a slave of instincts, drives, conditionings.
One is formed by heredity and environment, but one has the *imagination
of freedom*, or, as James calls it, "the illusion of freedom." In his old age,
James was prepared to live by that illusion.[26]

7 Gestalt Psychology: Psychophysical Isomorphism and Insight-Thinking

T his chapter has four objectives: first, to provide an overview of gestalt psychology's stand against elementalism; second, to consider the meaning and implications of "psychophysical isomorphism," the gestaltist model of the brain's structure and function; third, to comment on the evidence offered for and against the existence of insight-thinking and representational processes in apes; fourth, to survey the highlights of gestalt psychology's influence upon personality theory and social psychology.

Gestalt Psychology's Stand Against Elementalism

The unique feature of gestalt psychology, one that gives this school its special character, is its complete rejection of atomistic approaches to an understanding of behavior. Gestaltists hold that elementalism is the primary hazard of scientific method, philosophy, and art. One can become so careful in trying to specify variables and techniques as to lose the integrity of whatever he is investigating, communicating, or creating. A dilemma arises because human endeavor *without* specification of terms or techniques is confused and imprecise. Yet with excessive attention to terms or techniques, human endeavor becomes stilted, and only those issues for which concepts and methodologies already exist are treated. We no longer create; we just reproduce.

By now, reactions to the problems presented by elementalism are not new to us. We have seen how structuralism finally abandoned Fechner's grand attempt to describe consciousness in terms of its component sensations. We have seen how the mental mechanics of James Mill gave way to the mental chemistry of John Stuart Mill. We have seen how the reflexology of one-way dialectical materialism was forced to yield to the psychophysiology and higher-order conditioning of two-way dialectical materialism.

The only school, other than gestalt psychology, that did not have to overcome an initial predisposition toward elementalism is American functionalism. But the two schools are vastly different: Gestalt psychology's *exclusive* interest is to search out holistic phenomena which are especially illustrative of the fact that levels of organization cannot necessarily be equated with their entering components. Functionalism does not dispute the existence of these phenomena, although it reserves the right to question the gestaltist interpretation of them. Functionalism has broader interests than gestalt psychology. It is not so much against what gestalt psychology does as it is against any school's tendency toward giving what Woodworth long ago dubbed "marching orders." Thus, functionalism could absorb Fechner's psychophysical methods, Ebbinghaus's nonsense syllable technique, and Thorndike's puzzle box procedure, and continue to find meaningful use for all of them. Gestalt psychology, however, abandoned these experimental paradigms as being too unnatural. Watson and Pavlov were also dismissed for having modeled their views too closely upon stimulus-response reflexology. In the gestaltists' eyes the conditioners moved too quickly from observation of the rich and qualitatively different varieties of learning and perception to a restrictive quantitative analysis. Wolfgang Kohler drew the distinction this way:

Unfortunately, human interests tend to be so narrow that preoccupation with only the quantitative phase of research leads to . . . trouble. People who suffer from this ailment will soon fail to recognize problems which do not lend themselves at once to quantitative investigation. And yet, at the time such problems may be more essential and, in a deeper meaning of the word, scientific, than many purely quantitative questions.[1]

One can agree with Kohler, and even say "Bravo!" but refrain from committing the error of becoming too narrowly confined to qualitative problems of a special sort. Perhaps, in this respect, gestalt psychology has been overzealous and has been so since its very beginnings.

The year 1910 marked the arrival at the University of Frankfurt of three new assistant professors, Wolfgang Kohler, Max Wertheimer, and Kurt Koffka. Collectively, they were well-grounded in philosophy, physics, physiology, and mathematics. Each had his own theoretical and research concerns, but they developed a common, fervent mistrust of elementalism, regardless of the form of psychological inquiry in which it was manifested. Together, they founded gestalt psychology.

Every student of psychology is familiar with the counterelementalistic battle cry, "The whole is greater than the sum of its parts." However, this slogan is an erroneous version of the gestaltists' actual position. As noted by C.C. Pratt:

One phrase frequently associated with the unique properties of organized wholes was actually not used by the Gestalt psychologists, but nevertheless gave them no end of trouble: *The whole is more than the sum of its parts.* Many American psychologists were inclined to regard that statement as the quintessence of absurdity. Kohler often said that he wished his critics would remember that what he really said was that the whole if *different* from the sum of the parts.[2]

Kohler's statement pertains to the nature of reality. By asserting that the whole possesses its own inherent reality, the gestaltists made direct contact with the Kantian view that human beings possess an innate tendency to organize events. The gestaltists argued that reality is based upon perception, and that perception depended upon the bringing of an overriding coherence or organization to sensations, and to the stimuli evoking them.

Apparent Movement and Psychophysical Isomorphism

Max Wertheimer pursued the attack against elementalism through his research on apparent movement (or phenomenal movement; hence, "phi.") The problem that he examined (with Koffka and Kohler often serving as subjects) is one with which we all have at least a passing acquaintance through our going to the cinema. A motion picture film is composed of successive frames or stills that are passed rapidly through a beam of light, with the images focussed on a screen. Without giving it a second thought, we perceive *continuous* motion of the actors, actresses, and scenes in the movie, even though we are in fact seeing a series of *discrete* pictures.

The motion picture camera had not yet been perfected, but the stroboscope and tachistoscope were available to him. Wertheimer used these instruments to study parametrically the specific temporal and spatial conditions necessary to generate the illusion of real movement, from sequentially presented, *stationary* lights and objects. The "whole" was the organization by the viewer of apparent motion, from what were separate, static events. Successive, stationary events were pulled together by the viewer, and perceived as continuous, or real, movement.

Wertheimer's experiments resulted in the rejection of the then prevailing explanation of the perception of movement; namely, that the phenomenon depended upon sequential stimulation of the retina, and through the retina, the visual cortex. As noted by I.M. Spigel:

It is both tempting and convenient to give as a necessary condition for the perception of movement the successive stimulation of adjacent retinal loci. But any position which demands continuous displacement over a portion of the retinal mosaic as the necessary condition for movement perception is, to say the least, complicated by the existence of the phenomena of apparent movement. In the case of *phi* movement, for example, the appearance of continuous movement may be produced simply by the successive stimulation of discrete retinal loci, in the absence of continuous displacement of the stimulus upon the retina.[3]

Quite quickly, others identified a variety of visual, auditory, and tactual phenomena of a gestaltist character. Of the visual, a number did not require movement, and so have lent themselves to reproduction as figures in standard textbooks. (The Sander and the Muller-Lyer illusions are particularly compelling, and are shown in figure 7.1.) Collectively, they demanded something more than a wire model of the brain, and a brick-and-mortar idea of perception.

Thus, Wertheimer and his colleagues went a considerable step beyond that of the poet. They held that reality, and perhaps beauty too, are *not* in the eye of the beholder, but merely *begin* there. What we conceive as being "true" depends upon the organization we bring to sensations. The particular form of organ-

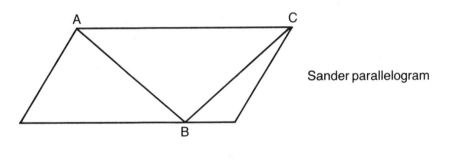

Sander parallelogram

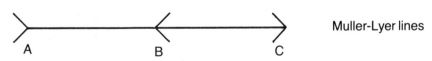

Muller-Lyer lines

Figure 7.1 The Sander and the Muller-Lyer illusions. In both cases, the distances AB and BC are equal.

ization, in turn, depends upon our momentary motivation and attention, upon our sensory organs, and—most important of all—upon the physics and processes of the brain. They urged that the linear-wire construct be replaced with a model taken from field physics, a discipline dealing with the lines of force generated by magnets and electrical currents. (Kohler had studied field physics under the eminent Max Planck). Thereby phi, as well as other organizational phenomena, could be explained. The model was eventually enunciated by Kohler as follows: "Psychological facts and the underlying events in the brain resemble each other in all their structural characteristics. Today, we call this the hypothesis of Psychophysical Isomorphism."[4] The implied *sameness of form* is that between the structure of psychological facts and the structure of physical events in the brain.

     Kohler's use of the word "structure" requires clarification. His argument was that the physical structure of an entity determines the functions possessed by that entity. Thus, when he employed the word "structure," he was subsuming as a necessary corollary what we ordinarily mean by the word "function" or "process." Some homely examples: (1) The cut and fabric of a flag are deliberately designed to determine the flag's characteristic motion in a breeze. (2) The presence of arcs on the legs of a chair is necessary to the back-and-forth, soothing motion of the ordinary rocker. (3) The molecular structure of water determines the fluidity of this substance. It also gives water its property of *dynamic equilibrium*, a term frequently used by Kohler in connection with psychophysical isomorphism. To elucidate: a pebble thrown into a pond causes ripples in the water, the molecules of which are at every instant in a state of changing equilibrium with respect to each other.

     Kohler's own example of dynamic equilibrium involves a metallic ellipsoid (i.e., an egg-shaped object) upon which electrical charges have been placed. The charges distribute themselves over the surface of this 3-dimensional volume conductor until a state of equilibrium is reached. No single charge on a spot on the surface of the ellipsoid can then be affected independently of the others. Disturb just one charge, and all other charges are influenced. Kohler then turned from electrostatics to electrical currents. He asserted:

Precisely the same is true of the steady states which currents assume when flowing in a network of wires, as also in larger continuous conducting media [i.e., wire networks, as well as surfaces and solids]. Everywhere in the system the intensity and direction of the local flow are such that the total distribution maintains itself unaltered. Again, therefore, one cannot understand what happens in a part of the conducting system without considering the distribution as a whole.[5]

Kohler chose the ellipsoid as an example because its shape is similar to that of the brain. He explained further: "Such examples have been introduced for a simple reason. What they tell us, we have to apply to the dynamic structures of the physiological processes in the brain, which are directly related to organized visual perception."[6]

The relation between psychophysical isomorphism and perception rests upon two interrelated syllogisms:

Syllogism 1
  a. The brain is a volume conductor of electrical charges.
  b. Volume conductors follow the rules of field physics.
  c. Therefore, the brain must follow the rules of field physics.

Syllogism 2
  a. Perception is dependent upon the brain.
  b. The brain follows the rules of field physics.
  c. Therefore, perception must follow the rules of field physics.

Kohler's research strategy was to concentrate on those cases of perception—e.g., apparent movement and other "illusions"—which he asserted could not be explained in terms of linear-wire models of the brain. He then offered interpretations in the language of field physics, and thereby implied that the brain—and of necessity, perception as well—followed the rules of field physics.

Before going further, it may help to understand Kohler's viewpoint if a familiar example is given of a solid object surrounded by a magnetic field. This will also enlighten us as to why he attached so much importance to field physics. We all learned in geography that our planet has a magnetic north pole and a "true" north pole, and that the navigator steers by a magnetized compass needle attracted to the former by a difference in polarity. The powerful attraction exists because the earth is surrounded by a magnetic flux which converges and is maximally dense at the top and bottom of the globe. Kohler's argument is that the structure and function of the brain—its anatomy and physiology—are such as to generate electrical currents through the *mass* of the brain. In addition, he held that the illusions studied by gestaltists proved the existence of these currents.

If the brain indeed acts as a volume conductor, then it should be surrounded by magnetic fields of force. Further, changes in visual stimulation at the eye should be accompanied by changes in these fields. In point of fact, investigators have been successful in detecting the existence of both these phenomena around the heads of human beings serving as subjects in visual research.[7] These results do not necessarily establish that *all* perceptual phenomena lend themselves to the gestaltist viewpoint. At present, it is safer to assume that depending upon circumstances, the brain functions either as a linear-wire system, a network-wire system, or a mass conductor, and that each of the three types of structure and function is of importance to perception.

Insight-thinking and Representational Processes in Apes

Kohler believed that "the whole is different from the sum of its parts" applied just as readily to thought, particularly to problem solving of the insight type, as it did to perception. His reason for asserting that there was a resemblance becomes clearer if we substitute the word "solution" for the word "whole," thus, "the *solution* is different from the sum of its parts." The "aha" phenomenon is experienced when we are able to transcend the properties of the individual components that enter into and constitute a problem, and are suddenly able to organize the solution.

We require still another step to understand the gestaltist's argument for relating thinking to perceiving, and Kohler helps us to take this step. In what may well have been his last formal lecture, "What is Thinking?" he discussed different usages of the term: (1) ". . . an inspection of memories" |e.g., I was thinking of our recent vacation|; (2) ". . . a synonym for having an intention" |e.g., I think I will go to lunch|. Of these first two types, he stated: "In both cases, the thinking involved is no particular achievement. It just refers to having mental contents, *in the absence of corresponding perceptual realities or actions.*"[8] (Note that Kohler did not bat an eyelash in taking it for granted that we are capable of *mentally representing* our perceptions of, and interactions with, the outside environment.) Kohler then discussed the third and most important usage of the term: (3) ". . . when thinking does become an achievement, that is, when it is productive. This happens when it changes our mental environment by solving problems which this environment offers. Now this is, of course, an entirely different story. . . . It is with thinking in this sense, with productive thinking, that I will . . . deal."[9] In other words, although all three types of thinking involve representational processes, the productive (or creative) type is the only one in which mental representations are changed during and by the very solutions they generate.

"Insight" is a special aspect of productive thinking. We infer insight if a problem is suddenly solved in the absence of changes in the *outside* world, and in the absence of overt trial-and-error approaches. Further, we infer that a change has occurred in the mental representation of the problem, and that the insight-solution to the problem will remain indefinitely with the organism.

In 1913, Kohler was given an opportunity to extend his research interests actively from the area of perceiving to the area of insight-thinking. The Prussian Academy of Sciences had named him director of the Anthropoid Station on the island of Tenerife in the Canaries, off the northwest coast of Africa. Because of World War I, Kohler stayed much longer than he had expected—a total of more than six years. His enforced sojourn gave him sufficient time for research, reflection, and writing to lead to his book, *The Mentality of Apes*. In this volume, he described his experiments with problem solving, using chimpanzees and other anthropoid apes as subjects. The two major classes of problems he studied are well known.

In one type, the animals had boxes of different sizes available to them. They were either to select one large box, or to assemble the right combination of smaller boxes and stack them, in order to climb up and reach a suspended banana. The chimpanzees displayed marked individual differences in their ability to solve the problem. Sultan, the smartest of his apes, did so quite readily. Rana, "a chimpanzee of particularly restricted intellectual gifts" was unable to do so, even after repeatedly watching Sultan.[10]

In the second type of problem, the chimpanzees had a number of hollow, bamboo sticks of different widths available to them. Each stick by itself was too short for the apes to reach a banana lying outside the experimental cage. They were required to select two sticks and, by inserting one into the wider opening of the other, make a single pole long enough to pull in the fruit. Sultan spent an hour in complete failure. He first tried using a single stick alone. He then tried pushing one stick with another toward the banana, but without joining the two. Finally, he arrived at the solution all at once. While squatting on a box, Sultan joined the two bamboo sticks, ran immediately to the bars of the cage, and reached out for the banana. Rana, however, never solved the problem.

Based upon the performance of his sample of chimpanzees, ranging in ability from Sultan to Rana, Kohler interpreted their behavior as indicating that at least the more gifted apes were quite capable of insight-thinking.

Soviet Refutation (or Is It?) of Insight-thinking in Apes

Kohler's work with insight-thinking in apes posed a serious challenge to the two-way dialectical-materialist tenet that only human beings possess productive or creative representational processes. For the Soviets, animal behavior, including that of higher apes, was to be understood entirely in terms of elementary conditioning phenomena, wherein productive thought has no autonomy and plays no part.

The experiments of Pavlov's student, E.G. Vatsuro, are directly germane to insight-thinking. He worked in Leningrad for nine years with a male chimpanzee named Rafael. Even before Vatsuro began this research (1937), biologists on the scene had already determined that Rafael could not solve the standing-on-a-box (or stacking-of-boxes) problem. The biologists found that "after unsuccessful attempts to obtain the reward from a height of two boxes, Rafael grabbed a third box and put it on his head!"[11] Vatsuro did not dispute their results, or their methodology.

As to the joined-stick problem, Vatsuro hypothesized that Kohler's chimpanzees did not really "solve" a problem that was new to them, let alone show insight. The situation was not novel, because the act of reaching out for an object with a branch to obtain a fruit is commonplace in their natural habitat, and readily generalizes to a stick in the laboratory. It is only in this sense that the chimpanzee can use a "tool"; the animal cannot fashion one, as superficially appears to be the case in the joining of two sticks. Vatsuro claimed that the joined-stick solution did not demonstrate either insight or tool-making, because of an artifact in Kohler's research design. Specifically, the visual-motor field to which the chimpanzees were exposed was severely restricted. Vatsuro believed he proved his point by having two phases to his own experiment. The phases differed in the extent to which the visual-motor field was limited.

Phase 1. During the first phase, Vatsuro gave Rafael two bamboo sticks of different diameters. By joining them, the ape could reach through the bars of the cage, and obtain a banana. It took two days for Rafael to succeed in the task, but he did not retain the solution. On the third day, the chimpanzee again tried to reach the banana with just one stick; only occasionally, when unsuccessful with the one stick, would he join the two, and pull in the banana.

Phase 2. After 10 days, Rafael was again given two sticks, one of which was modified as shown in figure 7.2. The wider of the two sticks was altered to have a junction of three side openings, in addition to the "natural" hole at the end of the stick. The latter opening was the only one which, when chosen, was effective in lengthening the narrower stick. Rafael tried numerous combinations, until he stumbled on the correct strategy for joining the two components. But after doing so, he did not attempt to reach the banana.

An analysis of Vatsuro's experiment first appeared in Polish, in Y.N. Dembovskii's *The Psychology of Apes*, published in the Soviet Union in 1963. A translation follows:

(1) The correct solution did not occur immediately; (2) repetition of the experiment did not evoke immediate reproduction of the previous solution; (3) Rafael joined the sticks even in the absence of the reward; (4) originally the sticks were joined without effectively lengthening the

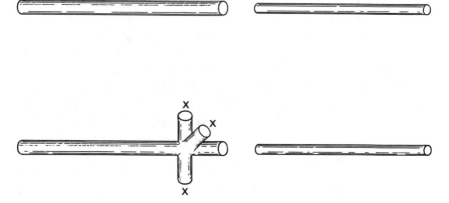

Figure 7.2 Kohler's and Vatsuro's versions of the joined-stick problem. In the latter case, insertion of the narrow stick into the side-openings (x), was not effective in making a single, long stick.

tool as a whole; (5) in the process of repeating the experiments, the animal, as a rule, repeated all the previous errors. All this does not indicate an intellectual solution of the task. The manipulation of the sticks cannot be considered a part of the whole process of food acquisition since it has its own stimulation. It may occur with the same success both with and without a reward. There is no doubt that the aim of manipulating the sticks is not to lengthen the stick. The ape's frequent errors even after the solution of the task indicate the absence of his comprehension of the situation.[12]

It is interesting to conjecture whether the multiple-opening, joined-stick problem could have been solved by Sultan, Kohler's brightest ape. Perhaps Vatsuro's Rafael was more like Rana, one of Kohler's less-gifted chimpanzees, than like Sultan. Striking individual differences in visual-motor organization exist among human beings. They may also exist in chimpanzees.[13]

Regarding Language in Apes

Research into whether chimpanzees are capable of a human type of thinking such as insight invariably raises the question of whether chimpanzees can be taught a human type of nonverbal language. Presumably this follows, because if the apes could be taught to communicate semantically with their experimenters, it would buttress the argument that they were capable of abstract or representational thinking.

The Russians demonstrated in the 1940s and early 1950s that apes could be taught to use sign-language (finger and arm signals) to *designate* different foods.[14] Their findings implied, however, that semantic or syntactic gestural language were beyond the ape's capacity. After surveying the results of his own extensive research at Columbia University, experiments in which the chimpanzees were trained to use hand signs to put "words" together, Terrace came to the same conclusion as the Russians: chimpanzees are not capable of putting together a sentence, or of following grammatical rules. The previously reported, appar-

ently successful efforts (including his own) accomplished nothing
more than having trained the apes to emit conditioned chains of
behavior.[15]

Regarding Cognition in Apes

Can chimpanzees or other higher apes think produc-
tively or creatively, as asserted by Kohler, notwithstanding their
apparent inability to generate syntactic language? Overall, do
chimpanzees possess cognition and consciousness even remotely
resembling that of the human being? A special issue of the journal *The Behavioral and Brain Sciences* was devoted to this second
broader question.[16] There were almost as many answers given as
there were author-commentators. Although he was not among the
contributors, W.A. Mason elsewhere provided the crispest reply to
date. He wrote:

Attributes such as "richness of associations," "reflective thought," "sym-
bolization," "images," and the like, so often cited as differentiating man
from ape, remain elusive and ill defined in the human case and can hardly
provide a firm basis for inter-species comparisons. To foreclose the issue now is to say, in effect, that the ape utterly lacks abilities and functions that have yet to be adequately described in ourselves.[17]

Koffka, and Back to Human Psychology

Of the three cofounders of gestalt psychology, Kurt
Koffka was the most daring in attempting to apply gestalt principles to problems of human behavior. He argued that the organizational rules of gestalt psychology, as established in perception,
are fundamental to an understanding of most other aspects of
human behavior, including personality and social psychology. In
a word, the way we perceive is basic to *all* behavior.

The steps leading to his position are suggested by

Woodworth and Sheehan's somewhat hesitant interpretation of Koffka's *Principles of Gestalt Psychology* (1935). The first step is one with which the reader is already familiar. We do not ordinarily respond directly to stimuli, but to our perception of them, i.e., to the way we organize sensations. Koffka drew a general distinction between the perceived (or—his term—"behavioral") environment versus the real (or physical) environment. The second step is this: the way we perceive stimuli depends upon field physics and their attendant organizational principles, as explored here in the discussion of psychophysical isomorphism. Third, the child's unfolding idea of self versus not-self depends upon the perception of qualitative differences between *outside*, exteroceptive stimuli (mainly visual and auditory) and *inside*, interoceptive stimuli (including tactual, proprioceptive, and internal sensations.) Fourth, the distinction between one's self, other such selves, and the environment is always in a state of flux or tension. The reason is: "The physical situation may be deceptive or at least difficult to grasp, our senses have their limits, and our desires may blind us to the real facts. Persons as well as things are not always what they seem."[18]

In summary, the point is that we become what we are on a personal basis, and act the way we do on an interpersonal basis, because of the way we perceive. And the way we perceive, in turn, is governed by the rules of gestaltist, organizational principles.

The Future Task of Gestalt Psychology?

Gestalt psychology has had the salutary effect of restraining behavioral scientists and therapists from oversimplifying their subject matter. By itself, that is a major contribution. As noted in the opening to this chapter, however, the gestaltists are not alone in their battle against an overly zealous elementalism.

But the gestalt school has accomplished more than a rejuvenation of mental chemistry. Investigators have demon-

strated previously unsuspected holistic phenomena within perception, and have established important theoretical connections
between perception and thought. Gestalt relations between perception on the one hand, and emotion, motivation, and purposivity on the other, undoubtedly also exist, as implied by Koffka. These
relations have not yet been as well formulated as those between
perceiving and thinking. Perhaps that is the future task of gestalt
psychology.

8 Freudian Psychoanalysis: Major Concepts and Their Relation to Conventional Variables

This chapter has two primary objectives: first, to provide a brief overview of the major constructs, principles, and therapeutic phenomena of Freudian psychoanalysis; second, to illustrate how the Freudian concepts and techniques are related to the variables of conventional psychology.[1]

The Uniqueness of Psychoanalytic Theory

Sigmund Freud's psychoanalytic theory differs from all other forms of psychological inquiry in this one crucial respect: the psychoanalytic movement had its beginnings in the therapist's office with attempts to help neurotics. As Freud pondered the problems of his patients, he formulated his theory. As he met with success or failure, he modified his theory. As he became more confident of his conceptions, he extended his theory, even to the point of application to "normal" persons.

The reasonably well-read individual who is curious about the sources of human behavior will sooner or later encounter ideas that are attributable to Freud. Although some knowledge on the reader's part of Freud's writings can therefore be taken for granted, we will review them briefly so that we might have a common point of departure. We reserve for the next chapter a general critique of both Freudian and neo-Freudian psychoanalysis. Our task now is to secure a knowledge of the basic psychoanalytic propositions, and to do so without bias or preconception. We begin our survey of psychoanalysis with definitions of Freud's major theoretical constructs.

Freud's Constructs

There are two categories of concepts in Freudian theory. The first describes levels of consciousness or awareness; the second, functional components of personality. For our purposes, personality is defined as an individual's characteristic modes of dealing with himself, with the world, and with the people in it.

Levels of consciousness: For Freud, there are three levels of consciousness—the conscious, the preconscious, and the unconscious. They are to be viewed as lying along a continuum of awareness. The *conscious* is that part of personality of which the individual is ordinarily aware. It includes his thoughts and feelings, especially those that he assumes to provide the basis of his activities. He can readily communicate these thoughts and feelings to others, as deemed necessary or desirable. The *preconscious* is that part of personality of which the individual is not aware at the moment. However, he can bring preconscious thoughts and feelings into awareness without great difficulty. The *unconscious* is that part of personality of which the individual is unaware, and which cannot be brought into awareness without assistance. Its contents either have never been conscious, or have been repressed—pushed back from awareness.

Functional components of personality: An individual's personality is comprised of three functional elements: the id, the ego, and the superego. The *id* consists of primitive asocial urges that demand immediate gratification. (The word "id" is a special use of the Latin *id*, meaning "it"; in turn, a translation of the Greek *es*, meaning "primal urge.")[2] The id is entirely unconscious. The *ego* mediates between the id's demands for immediate gratification and the requirements of reality. (The word "ego" is derived from the Latin *ego*, meaning "I"). The ego is partly conscious, partly preconscious, and partly unconsciousness. The *superego* exerts pressure on the ego to curb the desires of the id, and to feel guilty about gratification. It is generated from the rules initially laid down by the parents, and later by society in general. The superego is partly conscious, partly preconscious, but largely unconscious. It is because the superego is largely unconscious that it is not quite synonomous with the colloquial view of conscience. In the everyday conception of conscience, we have a little voice within us telling us what to do and what not to do. The superego does not provide such instruction, because of its mainly unconscious character. For example, if one is too conservative or rigid about certain demands of the id, he probably cannot implicitly or explicitly verbalize why; in fact, it is likely that he is unaware of that condition.

Freud believed that anxiety stemmed from the pressure brought upon the ego by the id, the superego, and the external world of reality. He wrote:

The proverb tells us that one cannot serve two masters. The poor ego has a still harder time of it; it has to serve three harsh masters, and has to do its best to reconcile the demands and claims of all three. These demands are always divergent and often seem quite incompatible; no wonder that the ego so frequently gives way under its task. The three tyrants are the external world, the superego, and the id. . . . The ego . . . feels itself hemmed in on three sides and threatened by three kinds of danger, towards which it reacts by developing anxiety when it is too hard pressed.[3]

Although Freud eventually elaborated upon his explanation of the sources of anxiety (for example, by indicating that the ego's *perception* of what is going on in the real world changes, because the ego itself keeps changing in response to imbalances from the opposing forces of the "tyrants"), the quoted statement remained central to his theory.

Freud's Principles

There are two major principles that account for the development of personality. They are the pleasure principle, and the reality principle.

Pleasure principle: This law begins to operate during infancy, when the id is virtually in entire command. It describes the early circumstances that lead to immediate physiological satisfaction. Pleasures, such as nourishment and cuddling, are brought to the infant. Aversive stimuli are removed or kept away. In its essentials, the pleasure principle is derived from a hedonistic, homeostatic model of stimulation, the steady or "normal" state of which is nonirritation, or even contentment. The principle operates by means of the *primary process, and continues doing so into adult life.* The primary process is quite a-rational; it draws no distinction between true and fantasized events, and is oblivious to the actual serial ordering of events in space or time. The primary process accordingly dominates during dreaming, when the pleasures sought in fantasy are expressed symbolically as wishes seeking fulfillment (latent content), and when events in time and space are rearranged, condensed, distorted, and even disguised (manifest content)—all to accommodate the underlying pleasure principle. However, the accommodation occurs within constraints imposed by the reality principle.

Reality principle: This law describes how the ego evolves as a consequence of the pressures brought upon the individual by the id, by the superego, and especially by the real world. The human being must learn to interact with his natural and cultural worlds in such a manner as to be more than a passive recipient of pleasures, and to do so in a manner that is amenable to society's conventions. To reach this state, the infant must first distinguish between mental representations or memory images of objects in the real world, and his immediate sensory experience of them. Therein lies a crucial difference between the id and the ego: "The basic distinction between the id and the ego is that the former knows only the subjective reality of the mind whereas the latter distinguishes between things in the mind and things in the external world."[4]

The reality principle governs the individual's growing awareness of the difference between mental imagery and sensory experience. It counters the pleasure principle to allow the person *actively* to seek returns in the real world, and even to plan or postpone gratification into the future. The reality principle operates upon the ego through the *secondary process*. "By means of the secondary process, the ego formulates a plan for the satisfaction of the [particular] need and then tests this plan, usually by some kind of action, in order to see whether or not it will work. . . . In order to perform its role efficiently the ego has control over all of the cognitive and intellectual functions; the higher mental processes are placed at the service of the secondary process."[5] It is important to note that although the ego *uses* cognition, the ego and cognitive processes are not equivalent. Freud's "I" is not to be confused with Descartes's "I" in "I think, therefore I am." To get the proper perspective, we need but recall Freud's comment concerning the ego's triad of masters.

Psychosexual Stages of Development

While the theory of psychosexual stages of development is important to Freudian doctrine in its own right, it also serves to illustrate the relation between the pleasure and reality principles. What Freud tried to do in formulating his hypotheses was to indicate where tensions between the two principles and their respective processes might arise and where removal of these tensions might take place.

If a person undergoes sequential changes in the source of sexual stimulation in a normal way (with the connotations of sexual being *extremely* broad), "The person becomes transformed from a pleasure-seeking, narcissistic infant into a reality-oriented, socialized adult."[6] According to Freud, the newborn infant can be stimulated and will have a pleasurable sensation more or less amorphously—in any area of his anatomy. This first stage is called the diffuse stage of psychosexual development. Touching the skin, brushing the hair, touching the toe or finger or stomach, just plain cuddling are pleasurable to the infant. Quickly, however, the major site of pleasure becomes the mouth, the lips, the buccal cavity. In this stage, the child is busy suckling and presumably derives most of his pleasure from oral contact. There is a transition at the end of 8 months (these time periods are not very specific) to the anal zone as the principal site of erogenous stimulation. The anal area remains the chief pleasure zone up until the age of about 2 or 3 years. This span of time corresponds to the toilet-training period in an individual's life. The type of pleasure involved is first an expulsion of feces, and then, as toilet training becomes effective, retention. Some time between the second and fourth years, the anal phase gradually gives way to the genital phase. Here the child finds his main source of pleasure in the stimulation of the genital area. Because of the child's obvious physiological unreadiness, and the social pressure conveyed by the repressive admonishments of parent, nurse, and other authoritarian figures, this phase gives way eventually to the latent phase. Although immature sexuality may be present in this stage, it goes dormant. It is during this latent stage of psychosexual development that the well-known Oedipus complex comes to the fore, with the boy being in love with his mother and repressing thoughts about the relationship; similarly, the girl is in love with her father.

Finally, the child becomes an adolescent, reaches puberty, and ordinarily makes a heterosexual adjustment, such that his or her pleasure comes from and with a member of the opposite sex.

Freud held that if the human goes through these stages of psychosexual development in a normal manner, no neurosis is possible. A neurosis develops when the individual becomes arrested or fixated at some particular stage of psychosexual development. This is not to imply, however, that the person may not reach heterosexuality and establish a lasting relationship with a member of the opposite sex. This can occur, and does occur, but with the neurotic individual unknowingly deriving an inordinate amount of satisfaction from some previous stage of psychosexual development. It is commonplace, for example, to read of someone's being fixated at the anal stage or having an anal personality. This does not usually imply any literal, physical involvement with the anal area. The fixation could take the form of preoccupation with matters of cleanliness or much concern with saving or hoarding material. This kind of person cannot throw anything out, and is inordinately retentive of possessions; or, on the contrary, is delighted to bring out his stamp collection and to exhibit their neat arrangement against the page. Such an individual would be "neurotic" in the sense that much of his energy is expended in what are essentially childish ways of coping with the environment and with other persons.

Therapeutic Phenomena

Freud was indebted to his early colleague, Joseph Breuer, for the idea of using the technique of free association, as a means whereby the contents of the unconscious could be revealed. Breuer was treating patients suffering from hysteria; i.e., a paralysis or a memory loss without neurological basis. Breuer routinely took case histories, with particular attention given to when the symptoms first were noted. He found that in many instances, the symptoms disappeared after the patient recounted the details of the circumstances surrounding the onset of the ailment. Breuer called this phenomenon *catharsis*, a "talking-out" or "purging." Unfortunately, catharsis afforded only temporary relief. Nonetheless, Freud was sufficiently impressed to elaborate upon his colleague's finding. He encouraged in his patients not only recollections associated with the origin of symptoms, but associations of *any* sort that came to mind. He found that his patients would, without deliberate instruction, recount childhood memories, including even those of their early dreams, to which in turn they would again volunteer associations. Freud's conviction grew stronger that the associations were not random, but existed for a reason. There was a cause behind each association. Further, he became certain that special importance should be attached to the contents of the patients' dreams, as well as to their associations to those contents. Between the two—the dreams and the associations to them—dream interpretation became possible. Thereby, he saw facets of their personalities that not only would otherwise have remained obscured, but which he considered to be essential to comprehending their problems.

The "royal road to the unconscious," as Freud called dream interpretation, can be found if the patient who has had the dream, and the analyst going over the dream plus its associations with him, can recognize the latent content, after examining the manifest or symbolic content. The reason why one can get at the unconscious through dream analysis is that, during sleep, the ego relaxes.

Figure 8.1 suggests why, at least in the Freudian system, dream interpretation is so important. It represents a crude way of tying together the functional components underlying psychoanalysis, and the behavior of the individual. To review, the id is largely unconscious and makes demands upon the person for

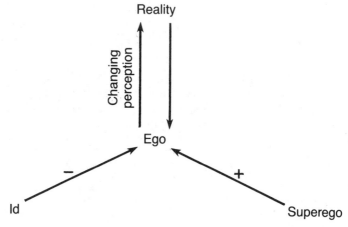

Figure 8.1 Diagram showing interaction among reality, ego, id, and superego. The ego's perception of reality changes during life.

immediate gratification. The ego filters these demands in terms of the dictates or requirements of a perceptually changing reality. The superego puts pressure on the ego in a direction opposite to that of the id. In the dream itself, the dictates of reality are partially discounted by the ego. Thereby the demands of the id and superego are able to come out to a greater extent. By looking at the demands of the largely unconscious id and superego, as revealed in dreams, the therapist can obtain a view of the dynamics of the patient's unconscious. These dynamics include repression, resistance, and transference.

The following definitions transmit the full Freudian flavor:

Repression is an unconscious exclusion from . . . consciousness of objectionable impulses, memories and ideas. The ego . . . acts as if the objectionable material were nonexistent. *Resistance* is a continuation of repression which interferes, often actively, with the progress of the analysis. It is an expression of the wish to maintain the repression of the unconscious desires. The analysis of the resistances, along with the analysis of the transference, forms the basic task of psychoanalysis. In *transference*, the patient generalizes his past emotional attachments to the analyst. . . . The analyst is a substitute for the parental figure. . . . In positive transference the patient loves the analyst and wishes to obtain love and emotional satisfaction from him. In negative transference the patient views the analyst as an unfair, unloving, rejecting parental figure and accuses him of all his parents' past injustices.[7]

The analyst working together with the patient interprets the patient's dreams and associations, to make clear the source of his often conflicting feelings toward the parental object, as well as other unconscious conflicts.

Note on the history of dream interpretation: The importance attached to dream interpretation hardly began with Freud. To realize this, one need but recall the biblical story of Joseph in the Land of Egypt. Indeed, D. Bakan has sought to relate Freud's emphasis upon dream analysis to the fact that Freud, when he was a child, was surrounded by some of the culture of the Jewish mystical tradition.[8] Bakan's hypothesis is that Freud was influenced by this early exposure and that his later emphasis upon dream analysis stems from some of the considerations which one finds written in the commentaries contained in the Talmud. Some of these statements are at least 2,000 years old. One scholar quoted in the Talmud clearly affirms the psychological origin of dreams, "A man is shown in a dream only what is suggested by his own thoughts." Another passage bears both on the sexual symbolism of dreams and on the Oedipus complex. A person reported "I saw myself in a dream, pouring oil on olives." The interpreter replied, "This man has outraged his mother."[9]

By way of contrast, this passage appeared in the first volume of the *American Journal of Psychology*, published in 1887–88:

There is a tendency to be interested in the matter of the dream, in its aesthetic effects, much as we react towards ideas and events of real life in relation to our well-being. Of course this is the unscientific stand-point. The fact that a person dreams much or little is of more significance than what he dreams. A curve representing the variations from day to day in the amount of dreaming has scientific interest, while the hobgoblins that we saw are of interest to children.[10]

Relations of Freudian Psychoanalysis to Conventional Variables

Psychoanalysis developed independently of but parallel with experimental psychology. Although the approaches were parallel, there are points of contact between the two. Such instances appear, however, to be almost coincidental. Certainly some psychologists are concerned with psychoanalytic research, but by and large the working psychologist in his laboratory has little interest in the testing of analytic hypotheses. Despite this lack of interest there are several striking resemblances between the analytic and the experimental approaches to understanding behavior. Perhaps these resemblances stem from the fact that both approaches are grounded in the belief that only a deterministic view of behavior will eventually lend itself to an accurate description of behavior.

One way in which the analytical approach and the experimental approach seem to have a common direction is in the attachment of importance to past experience. In the Freudian instance, it takes the form of emphasis upon child-rearing and the anxieties of the infant. In the case of learning theorists, it takes the form of asserting that the previous reinforcement history of the organism must be known if we are to understand the organism's current behavior. It is important to know the past reinforcement history of the subject because the same peripheral behavior may be established and shaped by quite different circumstances. Both the analyst and the experimentalist emphasize this point.

A second way in which the analyst and the experimentalist appear to see eye to eye is in the autoregulatory nature of drive reduction. Freud put it this way:

In the theory of psychoanalysis we have no hesitation in assuming that the course taken by mental events is automatically regulated by the pleasure principle. We believe, that is to say, that the course of those events is invariably set in motion by an unpleasurable tension, and that it takes a direction such that its final outcome coincides with the lowering of that tension—that is, with an avoidance of unpleasure or a production of pleasure.[11]

The essence of the foregoing quotation of Freud is quite similar in concept to the behaviorist's view that drive and reinforcement are defined as part of a loop system. Reinforcement does not have any empirical meaning independent of some prior operation which establishes a drive. In short, corresponding to the pleasure principle are the experimental concepts of reinforcement through drive reduction, and of adaptation models in general.

The primary process affords a third instance in which there is a point of contact between analytic theory and experimental psychology. The primary process refers to the phase in which the human infant acquires those patterns of behavior which are based upon immediate bodily satisfaction. There is, however, no infant-originating interaction with the environment. The individual is incapable at that stage of life of doing anything to influence the environment through behavior originating particularly with him. He cannot walk, he cannot talk; pleasures are brought to the infant, so to speak. The circumstances just described, those in which no action is taken by the organism upon the environment, are reminiscent of the situation that exists during Pavlovian conditioning. Here, one stimulus (the reinforcing stimulus) follows another stimulus (the initiating or conditioned stimulus) regardless of what the organism does. The learning that takes place is at the gut level, in that it involves autonomic modes of responding. The fact that much of our learning takes place in a classical sense, that is, autonomically, and takes place without words being tagged on as either stimuli or responses, has significant implications for problems of therapy.

Even as the modern-day psychologist distinguishes between two types of learning, classical and instrumental, so Freud found it necessary to distinguish between two psychoanalytic processes, the primary and the secondary. The primary process is the functional arm of the pleasure principle, and is probably related to classical conditioning; the secondary process (more broadly, the reality principle) is related to instrumental conditioning. According to the reality principle, reinforcement is obtained by the organism as a consequence of his action upon the environment, and to the modern-day psychologist, this is a simple statement of operant behavior. Freud's interest in the reality principle was the development of the ego. Recall that the ego, for Freud, is concerned with modifying the opposing demands of the id and the superego in keeping with the structure of the real world around the organism. In a learning theory sense, the ego consists of the correlations between the cues of the environment and the responses of the organism, the two being joined together by reinforcement contingencies.

The final example of a relation between psychoanalytic theory and experimental psychology consists of the concepts of repression on the one hand and avoidance behavior on the other. One of the tenets of psychoanalysis is the belief that the potentials of behavior can exist in an unaware state, known as the unconscious. The closest operational analog to this in experimental psychology lies in avoidance behavior. Some research has suggested that avoidance behavior can be induced in the laboratory with or *without* the subject's awareness.[12] The triggering-event can be either external or internal. In the latter case, it may be a symbolic representation—a thought, an ideation, or a feeling.

These points of contact between psychoanalytic and experimental theories have not been deliberately sought by either the experimental psychologist or the psychoanalyst. Their agreement can, however, be exaggerated. The central difference between the analytic and experimental theories still remains; the former is a conceptual system in which the principal ideas—particularly those pertaining to unconscious dynamics—are not readily amenable to controlled laboratory research. The experimental psychologist, on the other hand, attends to the need for an operational definition of his variables, so that he may work with these variables in the laboratory. Additionally, analytic doctrine is certainly oriented much more toward therapeutic needs than is the research of most experimental psychology. In recent years, however, there has been marked progress toward acceptance of what is therapeutically best for the patient, regardless of whether the source of the technique is psychoanalytic or experimental. We begin considering this reassessment by examining the neo-Freudians.

9 The Challenges to Psychoanalytic Theory and Therapy: Neo-Freudian and Behavioristic Dissent

No sooner did Freud formulate a coherent psycho-analytic theory, together with its systematic rules for therapy, then both came under attack. The challenges stemmed from within the psychoanalytic movement itself, as well as from outside. The objectives of this chapter are: first, to consider major dissent originating within the psychoanalytic movement; second, to offer a brief comparison and critique common to both Freudian and neo-Freudian forms of psychoanalysis; third, to comment on the challenge brought by the behavioristic movement; and fourth, to note the increasing eclecticism of psychotherapy.

Psychoanalytic Protest

The neo-Freudian psychoanalytic movement is not a unified reaction to classical psychoanalysis, as—for instance—Skinner's behaviorism was to functionalism. However, although it is diverse, the neo-Freudian protest does possess one general view: the rejection of Freud's emphasis upon the overriding importance of infantile sexuality. The downgrading of the idea that neurosis had its roots in the arrestment of sexual development was expressed in theoretical departures from Freud's conception of the structure (levels of consciousness) and of the functional components (id, ego, and superego) of personality. We will consider representative dissent, beginning with two of Freud's original disciples, Jung and Adler. As we shall see, they criticized classical psychoanalysis for quite different reasons, and developed their own conceptual systems.

Carl Gustav Jung and Analytical Psychology

Jung expanded on Freud's view of the nature and function of the unconscious. He theorized that human beings possess a collective, racially inherited unconscious, in addition to a personal one. Specifically, the collective unconscious is defined as follows:

The part of the unconscious composed of acquired traits and cultural patterns transmitted by heredity that is the foundation of the whole personality structure. It is universal, all men being essentially the same, is almost totally divorced from anything personal or individual, and is continuously accumulating memory traces as a result of man's repeated experiences. Archetypes are its structural components.[1]

The major archetypes are so pronounced as to transcend races, and to be present in the entire human species; others are specific to a given race.

More about archetypes in a moment, but first we have to confront the assumption that—because an unconscious representation of experience is present across races, or within a race—consideration *must* be given to biological inheritance. In point of fact, it is impossible from any anthropological viewpoint to counter successfully the direct, alternative explanation, namely, that the coexistent *customs* rather than the *genetics* of a race (however defined) are responsible for the presence of archetypes. In a word, we are dealing with a variation of the insoluable nature vs. nurture dispute—customs and genetics always go together. Since neither *extreme* position can be defended, we are better off setting aside the matter of whether the collective unconscious is indeed genetically determined. The issue is of no great moment in the larger context of Jung's intriguing ideas.

The concept of the archetype: There can be little doubt that all cultures have in common certain experiences that are repeated from generation to generation. Jung's idea of the "archetype" asserts that these repeated experiences gradually become incorporated, and lead to specific psychological tendencies that we all possess. "For example, since human beings have always had mothers, every infant is born with the predisposition to perceive and to react to a mother."[2] Chapter 1 indicated how this particular predisposition can be utilized to reify natural phenomena into the spirit known as "mother nature." For Jung, the development of spirits and animism is but a special case of the more general manifestation of archetypes. The chief archetypes, those that are of crucial psychological importance to the entire human species, are the persona, the anima-animus, and the shadow. He identified these three after considerable research into mythology. We shall return to the salience of the myth after considering the major archetypes.

Persona: The persona is the social mask worn by people. Its function is to hide the true person (the Jungian "self") from others. The persona is the role we play, one that is acted to create in others the opinion we wish them to have of us. We all find it necessary to hide ourselves to greater or lesser extent. We cannot, so to speak, bare our hearts as a way of life. We might be ashamed or victimized. The major risk presented by the persona, however, is that the ego (in Jungian psychology, "the conscious mind") may become so identified with the mask, that we lose contact with our true selves. Figure 9.1 shows how the self is influenced by the collective unconscious, the personal unconscious, and the ego. The "self" is deliberately depicted as a circle, a universal symbol known as "mandala," and believed to represent the striving for unity or oneness achieved through self-actualization. The persona is represented by the arrow going from the self to the ego.

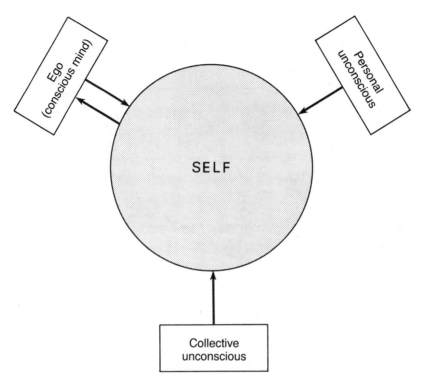

Figure 9.1 Representation of Jungian personality dynamics.

Anima-animus: It is well-known that the human being possesses both male and female biopsychological propensities. Of course, the one or the other ordinarily dominates. Jung held that there is enough of the male in the female, and vice versa, to form over generations an *idealized* conception (or archetype) in the human being of what to expect in the general behavior of a member of the opposite sex. For the man, the anima is the female archetype of his personality; for the woman, the animus is the male archetype. Misfortune befalls a love relationship if the archetypical expectancies held by either of the parties is seriously distorted.

The shadow: This archetype includes the residual of instinctual urges, originating from the human being's evolutionary descent from primitive ancestors. The shadow is quite asocial, and is given to aggression and gratification. When it infiltrates the ego (conscious mind), it can make one feel guilty about oneself, or—alternatively—cause one to perceive evil in others.

     Myth, metaphor, and imagery: Jung read *The Interpretation of Dreams* while he was experimenting with his word association test (see chapter 4). He gradually became convinced that the patterns (or *complexes*) of thought-feeling disruption which he detected by means of his test indicated a pervasive narrowness in Freud's conception of wish-fulfillment. Although Jung found that pleasure-related, psychosexual issues were indeed evidenced in the results of his test, and in his patients' dreams, they were quite subordinate to much deeper expressions of wishes, so deep as to transcend individual gratification, and to be indigenous to the human species as a whole. Accordingly, he formulated two hypotheses: first, that a culture's myths or legends should serve the same general purpose as that of an individual's dreams, namely, wish-fulfillment; second, myths of different cultures should possess in common the same symbolic representations of the major, fundamental wishes.

     As noted by Victor,

Many writers have pointed to similarities between dreams and legends. Roheim (1953) argued that they were not merely similar, but that most legends were derived from dreams. Jung's (1958) position was that some dreams are personalized legends; the same dynamics, derived from the racial unconscious, foster the creation of dreams by the individual and legends by the culture. Whatever their origins, we may infer that, in repeated retelling, the originator's idiosyncratic symbols have been replaced by common ones or have been adopted as symbols in their culture. By this development, the legend has been rendered suitable for its psychodynamic function.[3]

The same author elucidates on the relations among myth, metaphor, and imagery—all in the context of the utility of symbols in therapy. There may be

difficulty finding words to express thoughts for a number of reasons. Therapeutically significant fantasies are likely to be culturally taboo as well as individually conflict laden. In addition, there are prohibitions against uttering certain words. Theoretically, many early experiences occurred before the patient had developed language with which to represent them in memory and were encoded in physical (visual, tactile) images, to which words may later have become associated (Leavy 1973).

The lack of words to express an idea is exactly the type of situation that calls for a metaphor. . . . Both Leavy (1973) and Sharpe (1950) have argued that metaphor is the principal form of speech available for expressing unconscious imagery. For these reasons, and because every step in therapy involves a new revelation, formulation, or conceptual reorganization of associations, patients would seem to have a constant need for metaphors.[4]

Self-realization, individuation, and mid-life crisis: Unlike Freud, Jung postponed psychological maturity until about the age of 40. He maintained that by that time, *self-realization* (or *self-actualization,* the fulfillment of one's potentials) should be well on its way. However, self-realization cannot take place unless the influence of the archetypes and complexes is first recognized, understood, and reconciled. He called this process *individuation.* The term is hardly equivalent to exclusive concern for one's conscious ambitions, because Jung held that one cannot *become* one's self independently of a genuine regard for others, and a genuine acceptance of unconscious dynamics.

Jung drew attention to what is now called *mid-life crisis.* He found that

in the second half of life . . . many people are oppressed by a sense of futility and emptiness, and the need for something deeper and more significant. Jung's theory and practice were largely directed toward such people. . . . |H|e encouraged them to immerse themselves in mythology and to express themselves in some form of artistic activity. . . . |T|heir dreams also . . . were analyzed for indications of disturbing features, and for evidence of constructive stirrings of the unconscious pointing toward a degree of self-actualization. . . . Jung believed that the process of individuation was a slow one and that self-actualization was never completely achieved.[5]

Alfred Adler and Individual Psychology

Like Jung, Adler was one of Freud's original disciples. But over a ten-year period he contested Freud's ideas to the point where reconciliation became impossible. He resigned from the Psychoanalytic Society which he had helped Freud to establish, and started another organization. Within a year, this group had the title it bears today: The Society for Individual Psychology.

What was the fundamental nature of Adler's dispute with Freud? The answer is given in the very concept of the "individual." For Freud, the individual was a single entity, whose ego was determined by the id, the superego, and reality. For Jung, the individual was more of a social being, but at the expense of the self being influenced by a collective, in addition to a personal, unconscious. For Adler, the individual was more autonomous as a person—he could more *consciously* determine his own fate (hence, a critical distinction from Jung's idea of individuation and the influence of the personal unconscious); but concurrently (and as with Jung), the person was obliged to extend his interest in social matters.

Thus, the term "individual psychology" can be misleading if it is taken to connote an emphasis upon the separateness of one person from another. The interdependence among people must also be included in the concept, and given equal weight. If we realize Adler's position at the onset, that "One has to learn to feel so much part of other people that egoism becomes altruism and altruism contains also egoism,"[6] then we can begin to understand why he is known jointly for being both the father of ego psychology and a founder of social psychology.

Adler's model: Adler's model for the development of personality has the following steps, some of which interact with each other. They are elucidated here only as considered necessary. (1) *Experiences of infantile helplessness.* (2) *Subsequent feelings of inferiority.* (3) *Striving for superiority.* Here the child endeavors to overcome inferiority by striving toward goals that permit feelings of superiority. These goals include, but are by no means limited to, sexual attachments. (4) *Existence of guiding fictions.* This concept implies both goal-directedness as well as unrealistic aspirations. It is analogous to but goes beyond the later Freud's notion of the ego-ideal, "that part of the superego which carries the child's admiration for idealized parental figures . . . [and] results in the individual striving toward perfection by attempting to live up to the expectations or standards of the idealized parental figures."[7] The concept of guiding fiction is broader than that of ego-ideal, because it is not limited to the exclusive influence of idealized parental figures, but extends to the influence of society in general. (5) *Creative self.* The creative self begins emerging at about five years of ago. It derives its name from how a person creates the world around him, including his guiding fictions. One function of the creative self is similar to that indicated by the "perceptual" arrow in figure 8.1. However, this function alone is quite insufficient to convey Adler's notion of the self taking responsibility for its own destiny. The creative self becomes capable of controlling its own future, to the extent that it is formulated both through a growing awareness of personal autonomy and through an increasing manifestation of social interest. (6) *Style of life.* The start of a person's life style ("characteristic mode of living . . . , of the way . . . he pursues his goals")[8] coincides with the emergence of the creative self. It is a critical stage, for if a child is either pampered or neglected too much, he will not develop social interests in a normal fashion. The tendency is for such people subsequently to withdraw from social interaction "into a world of pretense and illusion."[9] They do so at the eventual expense of their own self-esteem, and the esteem with which others hold them.

Whereas Freudian psychoanalysis seemingly dooms the adult on the basis of how his fate was determined during infancy and early childhood, Adlerian individual psychology appears to offer more hope. The joint needs of expressing one's self and of meeting social responsibilities can only be satisfied if a person keeps looking forward toward his goals, and not backward toward circumstances over which he had little if any control. Adler identified the three major goals which he held we all strive for: effective community living, occupational fulfillment, and contented love and marriage.

Sullivan and Interpersonal Theory

Harry Stack Sullivan was probably the most influential of the founders of interpersonal theory. His position is that the concept of the "individual"—if taken as a singular, isolated entity—is a meaningless abstraction in theory and in therapy. An individual exists only on an interpersonal basis. Even one's perception of who he is as an individual (what Sullivan called the *self-system*), is based upon interpersonal relations. The self-system consists of habits that are acquired through interpersonal reinforcement contingencies, starting with the mother-infant relationship. These habits cultivate self-perceptions of a "good-me" (follows rules), "bad-me" (breaks rules), and "not-me" (dissociation because of infantile terror or disgust).[10] The different "me's" originate as ways of coping with anxiety resulting from threats to one's interpersonal security.

Sullivan was also concerned with impressions or attributions of causality. He held that there are three successively developed modes of organizing experience. The first is *prototaxic*, and operates during early infancy. In this stage there is no notion of causality because there is no structuring of experience in space or time. All is a welter of sensory confusion, both inside and outside the organism. The second mode is *parataxic*, and emerges later in infancy. Here, events tend to become associated in time and space, but only with regard to impressions of their serial order. Hence, the infant cannot draw any logical inference of causality. All he can "deduce" is that one event precedes another with a high degree of regularity. However, this limitation does not stop the infant from behaving as if the first event were the "cause" of the second—the "reason" for its existence.

Sullivan's ideas are in accord with the treatment given to associations and to logical inference in chapter 4. We noted then that seriality by itself can be deceiving, and that even the rules for drawing logical inferences of causality (e.g., J.S. Mill's methods of agreement and of difference) are fallible. Sullivan introduced the same canons through what he termed the *syntaxic*, or mature way of organizing experience. In this mode, the person attends to more than seriality in drawing conclusions concerning causality. He does this in an interpersonal, not a philosophical or laboratory context. Instead of depending upon logic, or laboratory replication and sampling procedures to establish that A is the cause of B, that the two are more than casually or wishfully connected, the individual depends upon what Sullivan called *consensual validation*. By falling back upon group opinion for reassurance, the individual avoids what might be misperceptions, personal biases, or ordinary superstitions. However, he does so at the risk of possibly accepting a false group opinion, while abandoning his own, correct one.[11]

Sullivan argued that parataxic thinking is characteristic of dreams and of disordered behavior. More importantly, he held that we are all occasionally prone to drawing parataxic inferences, regardless of our best efforts to the contrary. The role of the friend, or teacher, or clergyman, or therapist is to observe and to question both our assumptions and our conclusions. In a word, they participate in our customary interactions with the world, and with the people in it (Sullivan's *participant observer*).

Brief Critique of Psychoanalytic Approaches

Although the various psychoanalytic schools utilize different metaphors, they possess in common the following tendencies: (1) To reify psychological phenomena. Examples are Freud's id, Jung's shadow, Adler's creative self, and Sullivan's self-system. (2) To describe psychological processes in terms of oppositional polarities. Examples are: id vs. superego, anima vs. animus, inferiority vs. superiority, good-me vs. bad-me. (3) To assert claims for an exclusive understanding of human behavior, and to reject the approach of every other. (4) To accept the premise that all behavior is determined, while rejecting the experimenter's demand that the entering variables be operationally or statistically isolatable. Perhaps this inconsistency accounts for the following episode involving Freud. The incident was related by Roy Grinker, past president of the American Psychoanalytic Association: "I can remember full well when studying with him in Vienna that he angrily threw to the floor a letter he had received from Sol Rosenzweig, who was then studying at Harvard. Rosenzweig wanted to utilize psychoanalytic concepts experimentally in order to test the theory of repression. Freud angrily threw this letter away, saying, 'Psychoanalysis needs no experimental proof.' "[12] Freud may have felt that even if psychoanalysis *is* mainly a metaphorical model, it nonetheless is founded upon determinism. The one does not preclude the other. He therefore held that psychoanalysis follows the laws of causation, regardless of whether the model did or did not contain features that were amenable to the rules of empirical research. Indeed, Jung went so far as to assert that by its very nature, the unconscious was inaccessible to experimental analysis, "for the unconscious cannot be represented in terms of thinking or reasoning."[13]

While the psychoanalysts were taking each other to task, the main challenge to their collective viewpoint quite naturally came from the behaviorists.

Behavioristic Protest

Behavior therapy has its roots in the animal laboratory, which—in turn—owed its existence to Darwin's theory of evolution. The reasoning underlying behavior therapy is roughly as follows: (1) much of human behavior can be simulated in the laboratory by means of conditioning procedures in which lower forms of animal life are used as subjects; (2) conditioning procedures can be employed to produce in animals the kind of behavior that we call "neurotic" and "psychotic" when observed in human beings.

In 1927, Pavlov did not hesitate to use the words "acute neurosis" in describing the behavior of a dog which had been required to make too keen a discrimination between circles and nearly circular ellipses. Selection of the former was followed by food; choice of the latter went unreinforced (method of contrasts). "After awhile, [the dog] became violent, bit the apparatus, whined, and barked."[14] The implication is that human beings, just as dogs, develop neuroses when natural or social reinforcement contingencies require them to make too many fine discriminations.

In 1941, W. Estes and Skinner used the word "anxiety" with similar boldness in describing the decrease in rate of bar-pressing for food attendant upon a rat's being exposed to presentations of a five-minute tone signaling the impending arrival of a momentary, unavoidable shock to the paws. During the anxiety period, the rats defecated and became aggressive. The generalization was made to human behavior as follows: "psychological clinics are filled with cases of morbid and obsessive anxieties which are clearly the outcome of disciplinary and social training overburdened with threats of punishment."[15]

When we add to the foregoing the propositions that the occurrence of neurosis can often be ascribed to the acquisition of poor habits of adjustment, and that these detrimental habits can be diminished in strength and replaced with more adaptive habits, we have the essence of the behaviorist's approach to therapy.[16]

Of course, this approach was grounded in the philosophical conviction that the therapist should not get involved in the patient's cognitive, purposive, or affective attributes, since the existence of these attributes could only be inferred from outward behavior. The therapist was to avoid taking explanatory recourse to all unobservable qualities, because they were epiphenomena. He was to rely only upon directly observable behavior. That mandate precluded the explanatory utility of any notion of the unconscious.

The trend toward eclecticism, or nouns need not be demons: A central theoretical issue that has divided psychoanalysts and behavior theorists in the past is the charge that psychoanalysis is a modern version of demonology. The purported demon is the unconscious, with its active intrusion upon the behavior of the individual. Is the charge valid? Not when it comes down to general consideration of therapeutic practice. What the analyst perceives as active intrusion by the unconscious, the behaviorist perceives as counter control or behavioral nonresponsiveness by the patient. Neither kind of therapist falls back upon devils, whether of the unconscious or behavioristic variety, but both *necessarily* engage in the ancient practice of reification. For purposes of communication with the patient, both find it convenient to use nouns rather than verbs to describe patterns of thought, feeling, and action[17] (see chapter 6, p. 121). The one talks of the "unconscious"; the other, of "behavior occurring outside of awareness." Thus, the analyst presents his notion of repression in terms of the action of the unconscious; the behaviorist, in terms of unaware avoidance behaviors. For the one, resistance is a sophisticated extension of repression; for the other, a sophisticated extension of undetected, unaware avoidance behaviors. These extended avoidance behaviors are employed to preclude the recognition of, and thereby to strengthen the persistence of, routine avoidance responses. (This persistence is otherwise known in the field of conditioning as *resistance* to extinction!)

By now, behavior therapists, too, have encountered the occurrence of patient defiance, and have endeavored to develop strategies to cope with it.

It is easy to offer various post hoc explanations according to learning principles, but it is obviously useless to do so in terms of their predictive value. When examining therapeutic failures, to insist that target behaviors did not shift in a desired direction because the maintaining conditions and requisite reinforcements were inadequately manipulated, may be true in many instances, but this reasoning becomes tautological when consistently invoked as an explanatory principle.[18]

Conclusion

And here we must halt, for to continue leads us into issues of psychopathology and psychotherapy that are well beyond the scope of this work. Fortunately, we can conclude on a note of optimism: psychoanalysts and learning theorists are becoming increasingly receptive to the use of each other's concepts and practices. (The interested reader is referred to Marmor and Woods 1980, and Wolman 1983.)[19] The major reason is that each group (and those falling in between the two extremes) has had to acknowledge both its own failures as well as the other group's successes, and to search out the causes. Constructive reevaluation is in the air. These reassessments are fostering an eclecticism that draws upon the strengths of each approach. Even though the pace may not be constant, there is every indication that this forward movement will be maintained.

10 Epilogue and Prologue: Four Enduring Issues, and the Future of Psychology

The final chapter has two objectives. The first is to organize and to consolidate the contents of the book, through identification of "Four Enduring Issues." These are concerns about human nature that have persisted down through the ages. They encompass fundamental problems which have fascinated and frustrated each generation of philosophers, scientists, clinicians, artists, writers, and ordinary people. The second aim is to comment on the future of psychology.

Four Enduring Issues

The first issue is this: How do we humans reach the conclusion that a causal relationship exists between two events, or among a set of events? We began wondering about this problem right from the start, when we speculated about primeval man's perception of his world. We conjectured that his cognitive mode of organizing experience was largely parataxic—a perception of serial associations based upon temporal contiguity and spatial proximity of events; with the first event being considered the "reason" for the second; the second, for the third; and so on. Primitive man's way of organizing the world about him, and his own experiences in it was seen as a-logical and impressionistic.

Is it an exaggeration to assert that in our day-by-day living, we moderns are often quick to perceive causal relations (including interpersonal ones) in the same parataxic way as did primeval man? Of course, our schooling exposes us to associationism's rules of logic, and to positivism's rules of scientific method. Psychology teaches us further understanding by way of the rules of conditioning, of linguistics, of group behavior, and of perception itself. But we are here concerned with the way we perceive relationships, and infer causality *in our ordinary, daily existence.* The dramatic departure from logic is easy to spot; the routine departure is not.

And is it too much to declare that it is not necessarily a bad thing if we are not logical or scientific in all matters affecting our lives? Indeed, perhaps this is the lesson that poetry, art, and music teach. And even ethics—for doing the ethical thing is not necessarily the same as doing the scientifically logical thing, and this may be the lesson that religion teaches.

The second enduring issue follows from the first: Once we deduce that there is a causal relation between events, once we have satisfied that Kantian impulse to organize matters, then we are driven to find out the "why" of causality. We seek an explanation of *why* A occurred in the first place, to cause B. The *"how"* of A causing B is a separate matter, one leading to questions of elementalism and holism, to which we shall return. The seeking of the *why* of causes, or the *cause* of causes leads to the paradox of infinite causation. This paradox had to be "resolved" through the principle of finite causation in order for science to progress, otherwise we would have been immobilized in the laboratory. For many scientific matters, we are content with specifying "why" by pointing to the independent variables we introduce into an experiment. For other scientific matters, such a resolution is insufficient or impossible. We have seen that this is especially the case when trains of events appear to be self-initiating. They seem to initiate and to maintain themselves without an externally identifiable agent or cause. We then look *within* the entity or process being observed for an explanation. Almost inexorably, we are drawn into the maelstrom of "purpose," of an internally motivating force or agent, that seeks to accomplish a goal. At first, psychologists

(James and McDougall) used goal-direction or purposivism as a criterion for separating living from nonliving systems, but today we are not so sure. Self-regulating systems and computers have raised ancient questions concerning intentionality.

We have studied manifestations of this enduring issue while considering animism (spirits), functionalism (goal direction and "marks of intelligence"), behaviorism (Skinner's "homunculi"), Soviet two-way dialectical materialism (the human as a social activist, and the autonomy of higher-order conditioning processes), and psychoanalysis (unconscious motivation).

The perception of causality leads not only to questions of *origin*, or of *why*, but also to questions of manner, or of *how* one event causes another. *The third enduring issue* pertains to the relation between the structure and function of both living and nonliving systems, or to the *how* of a system's behavior. In the context of systems analysis, Kohler reminded us that living systems, just as nonliving systems, must follow physical and chemical laws. In this universal, law-abiding sense, we can say that God is a cosmologist. He draws no distinction between the living and the nonliving. It goes without saying, however, that Kohler would hardly have argued that the behavior of living systems can be *reduced* to physical and chemical components. Material components are necessary, but certainly not sufficient, contributors to living systems.

The Russian psychophysiologists have probably accomplished more along lines of examining the structure and function underlying behavior than any other group. They have kept an eye on the anatomy and physiology of the *entire* organism. They have not, in Woodworth's terms, made a "fetish of the brain," as perhaps did Kohler himself.

Soviet interest in psychophysiology is mentioned only to illustrate the main point concerning the *how* of behavior. It is this: the scientist is always caught between two "vectors." The one which directs him to specify variables, and to manipulate them carefully; and the other which directs him to retain the integrity of the phenomenon under investigation, and not to lose it in the very process of specification and manipulation. This tension is evident in almost every form of psychological inquiry: structuralism's *elements* of consciousness vs. the *whole* of consciousness; associationism's mental mechanics vs. mental chemistry; Russian one-way vs. two-way dialectical materialism (or reflexology vs. psychophysiology); traditional behaviorism's concentration upon action vs. radical behaviorism's extensions to thoughts and feelings; classical Freudian rigidity of theory and therapy vs. neo-Freudian flexibility; and mostly, of course, within the phenomena explored by the gestaltists—apparent movement, insight, and so forth.

The final enduring issue is this: The crucial question confronting each and every human being is one of personal existence, of identity, of "W*ho am* I?"

We have speculated that primeval man did not draw too sharp a distinction between the quality of identity *he* possessed, and the kind possessed by other entities of his universe. Such an outlook is essentially cosmological, and is formally represented in modern Hindu philosophy and religion.

The question "Who am I?" leads inevitably to the question "What is real?" for we cannot understand *personal* being—or personal reality—without grappling with the puzzle of general reality.

For psychologists, the problem of specifying reality becomes translated into one of mind-body dualism. Does the mind (or ideas) constitute reality, or is it the body (or matter)? Drawing mainly upon Plato's idealism and Descartes's interactionism, the structuralists attempted to specify personal identity by relating the psychological world of consciousness to the physical world of matter. Hence, the structuralist's psychophysical methodology, which remains as an important heritage to modern psychology. Similarly, the British associationists did much to enlighten us as to how feelings and thoughts emerge as a consequence of contiguities. In modern times, the Russians have turned contiguity into conditioning, thereby allowing them—through higher-order conditioning—to relate (but not reduce) the emergence of thoughts and feelings to materialism, as represented by anatomy and physiology.

The gestaltist way of tying together mind and body is best articulated in Kohler's principles of psychophysical isomorphism. The human perceives and thinks as a particular *kind* of being, because of the biophysical peculiarities of his brain.

Freud drew attention to the unfolding of each person's ego, or "I." He ascribed particular importance to the stages of psychosexual development, and to the conflicting influences of the id, the superego, and reality. Through his statement of the pleasure and reality principles (primary and secondary processes), Freud gave us a greatly expanded view of mind-body dualism. The neo-Freudians continued this broadening trend by emphasizing the part that other persons play in the emergence of an individual's conscious and unconscious aspects of "I."

Is the enduring issue "Who am I" more metaphysical than psychological? We respond "No."

Certainly, the question of *ultimate* reality *is* metaphysical in nature. But the rules and means whereby persons perceive their own identity, or their being, are psychological in character, and should not be dismissed as metaphysics. We have been enlightened by the continuing attempts of psychologists to comprehend the emergence and maintenance of individuality, whether within an experimental or a therapeutic context.

So the four issues that seem to have influenced psychology most, and still do in one way or another are these:

1. The perception of the relationship between events, or of causality—the problem of the mixture of the logical and the impressionistic ways in which we organize the inner and outer worlds of experience.

2. The concept of purpose, and how best to use this concept as an explanatory parameter, without falling to circular reasoning.

3. The tension between elementalism vs. holistic integration, as evidenced by the way we inquire into the structure and function of systems.

4. The problem of personhood, of how the "I" becomes established and maintains its particular identity.

Future: Perspective and Pitfalls

The future of psychology is bright, as long as we do more than merely develop new techniques and gather new facts. We must also remember to keep them in perspective. We can do so through continually reevaluating the past in light of our present discoveries.

There are two major pitfalls that lie in the path of achieving perspective. The first is to neglect the need to maintain psychology as its own enterprise. Although philosophy, biology, chemistry, and computer science can assist us in our search for psychological understanding, we must not forget the uniqueness of our subject matter. Along these lines, the psychoanalyst Silvano Arieti has commented on the logical problems that arise in attempting to reduce the mind and its functions to the brain. He called our times the Age of Pessimism, and stated as follows:

I am inclined to believe that the profound sources of pessimism and meaninglessness |characteristic of our times| have to be traced back to the modern philosophy of Western culture, which gradually has entered into popular culture and social habits. Unbelievable as it may seem, it started with the rejection of Cartesian dualism. According to many thinkers, there is no basic difference between mind and organism, psyche and soma, soul and body, the psychological and the physical. As a matter of fact, Descartes has become the common target of philosophical arrows. He is reputed by many to be the one who has plagued the modern world with dualism. . . . There is no doubt that to be human we need a human brain. But the human brain permits the emergence of something new which is not inherent in whatever preceded its appearance. The new level which emerges is so revolutionary, so different from the previous ones as to introduce a duality in the universe. The new level opens up the realms of infinite symbolization, imagination, fantasy, choice, freedom, commitment, autonomy, creativity, art, science, and psychosis—human functions or conditions which cannot be reduced to materialistic monism.[1]

The second pitfall is intolerance. Schools of psychology, types of experiments within psychology, the subdisciplines of psychology, altogether too often reflect an intolerance toward each other that is reminiscent more of ecclesiastical rectitude than of scientific endeavor. The reason is plain: the particular field of psychology (or of any other specialty in which we are trained) quickly becomes part of our *selves*, part of our fundamental outlook upon reality. Thus, any challenge to the basic assumptions of our field—whatever it may be—becomes a personal threat to us as *individuals*. We need not belabor the point, but it is just as easy to give lip service to intellectual tolerance as it is to religious or racial tolerance.

Hence, I have given repeated admonitions throughout this work to keep open-minded, to avoid academic smuggery, and to challenge the accepted doctrine or fact.

Notes

1. Cosmology, Spirits, and Animism: Origins and Continuing Influence

1. J.E. Pfeiffer, *The Emergence of Man* (1972), pp. 171–77.

2. Excerpted from an editorial appearing in the *Hindustan Times* (New Delhi), August 19, 1976, quoting R. Carrington's *A Guide to Earth History* (1956).

3. G.S. Brett, A *History of Psychology: Ancient and Patristic* (1912), vol. 1, p. 17.

4. B.B. Wolman, personal communication.

5. In this regard, J.J. Jaynes has advanced the idea that man did not develop consciousness as we know it, until the left (or language) side of the brain became more active. While compatible, the present analysis does not depend upon this intriguing argument. See J.J. Jaynes, *The Origin of Consciousness in the Breakdown of the Bicameral Mind* (1977).

6. Pfeiffer (1972), p. 189.

7. *World Almanac & Book of Facts* (1984).

8. Pfeiffer, p. 227.

9. A. Marshack, *Ice Age Art: 35,000–10,000 B.C.* (1978). Brochure describing an assembled collection which was exhibited at the American Museum of Natural History, N.Y. (May 24, 1978 to January 15, 1979).

10. Ibid.

11. Ibid.

12. S. Freud, *Moses and Monotheism*, in J. Strachey, ed., *The Complete Psychological Works of Sigmund Freud* (1964), vol. 23. pp. 80–92. The reference summarizes Freud's earlier work, *Totem and Taboo*.

13. S. Freud, *Totem and Taboo*, in A.A. Brill, ed. *Basic Writings of Sigmund Freud* (1938), p. 925. The statement attributed to J.G. Frazer is taken from his *The Golden Bough*.

14. In defending his position in 1938, Freud wrote: "In 1912 I attempted, in my *Totem and Taboo*, to reconstruct the ancient situation from which these consequences followed. In doing so, I made use of some theoretical ideas put forward by Darwin, Atkinson and particularly by Robertson Smith, and combined them with the findings and indications derived from psycho-analysis. From Darwin I borrowed the hypothesis that human beings originally lived in small hordes . . . under the despotic rule of an older male. From Atkinson I took . . . the idea that this patriarchal system ended in a rebellion by the sons. . . . Basing myself on Robertson Smith's totem theory, . . . I assumed that . . . the victorious brothers renounced the women on whose account they had . . . killed their father . . . and instituted exogamy. . . . The conformity between Robertson Smith's totem meal and the Christian Lord's Supper had struck a number of writers before me.

"To this day I hold firmly to this construction. I have repeatedly met with violent reproaches for not having altered my opinions in later editions of my book in spite of the fact that more recent ethnologists have unanimously rejected Robertson Smith's hypotheses and have in part brought forward other, totally divergent theories. I may say in reply that these ostensible advances are well known to me. But I have not been convinced either of the correctness of these innovations or of Robertson Smith's errors. A denial is not a refutation, an innovation is not necessarily an advance. Above all, however, I am not an ethnologist but a psycho-analyst. I had a right to take out of ethnological literature what I might need for the work of analysis" (Strachey [1964], vol. 23, pp. 130–31).

2. Structuralism: Ancient and Modern Mind-Body Dualisms

1. *The Complete Works of Homer* (1950), pp. vi–vii. The quotation is from the Introduction, which was written by Gilbert Highet. For a succinct account in modern English, see D.J. Hartzell, *Odysseus: The Complete Adventures* (1978).

2. W. Durant, *The Story of Philosophy* (1926), p. 20.

3. B. Weintraub, *New York Times*, September 18, 1974.

4. *Random House Dictionary of the English Language, Unabridged* (1967).

5. E. Heidbreder, *Seven Psychologies* (1932), pp. 28–29 (emphasis in original).

6. Robinson referred to him as a "modest materialist" because even though the soul held sway, Descartes did not ignore the physical reality that lay outside. D.N. Robinson, *The Enlightened Machine* (1980).

7. Durant, *Story of Philosophy*, pp. 382–83.

8. R.S. Woodworth, *Experimental Psychology* (1938), p. 450.

9. E.B. Titchener, *An Outline of Psychology* (1896), pp. 9–11.

10. G. Murphy, *Historical Introduction to Modern Psychology* (1949), pp. 84–91.

11. By working backwards, so to speak, the behavioral scientist obtains some empirical measure of sensation level, and plots sensation values as a function of stimulus values. If semi-log paper is used, then the logarithm form of the sensation curve is converted into a straight line. The slope of the line and its y-intercept yield the constants of the hypothesized integration.

12. Titchner, *Outline*, p. 67.

13. G.A. Miller, *Mathematics and Psychology* (1964), p. 100. If sensation levels are plotted as a function of stimulus values using log-log paper, and if a straight line is obtained, then a power relationship may be inferred.

14. D. Schultz, *A History of Modern Psychology* (3d ed., 1981), p. 66.

15. F.S. Keller and W.N. Schoenfeld, *Principles of Psychology* (1950).

16. H.S. Langfeld, "A Response Interpretation of Consciousness" (1931), p. 93.

17. C.T. Tart, "States of Consciousness and State-Specific Sciences" (1972).

18. E.R. Hilgard, "Consciousness in Contemporary Psychology," in M.R. Rosenzweig and L.W. Porter, eds., *Annual Review of Psychology* (1980), p. 15.

19. Ibid., p. 15.

20. A.H. Maslow, "A Philosophy of Psychology: The Need for a Mature Science of Human Nature," in F.T. Severin, ed., *Humanistic Viewpoints in Psychology* (1965).

3. Functionalism: Goal-Direction, Purpose, Feedback Theory, and Feedback Research

1. R.S. Woodworth, "Dynamic Psychology," in C. Murchison, ed., *Psychologies of 1930* (1930), p. 177.

2. W. James, *The Principles of Psychology* (1890), excerpted in R.J. Herrnstein and E.G. Boring, eds., *A Source Book in the History of Psychology* (1968), pp. 609–10 (emphasis in original).

3. W. McDougall, *Outline of Psychology* (1923), excerpted in Herrstein and Boring, eds. *Source Book*, pp. 615–18. "[McDougall] provides . . . an intermediate position between a conscious functional psychology . . . and a nonconscious behaviorism" (p. 615).

4. A. Rosenblueth, N. Wiener, and J. Bigelow, "Behavior, Purpose, and Teleology," in J.M. Notterman, ed., *Readings in Behavior* (1970), p. 47 (emphasis added).

5. E. Nagel, "Self Regulation," in D. Flanagan, ed., *Automatic Control* (1955), p. 2.

6. J.M. Notterman, *Behavior: A Systematic Approach* (1970), p. 55.

7. N. Wiener, *Cybernetics* (1948), p. 14.

8. J.M. Notterman, "Discussion of 'On-line Computers in the Animal Laboratory' " (1973).

9. J.M. Notterman and D.R. Tufano, "Variables Influencing Outflow-Inflow Interpretations of Tracking Performance" (1980). See also J.S. Hrapsky, "Effects of Training in Visual Observation upon Subsequent Visual-Motor Performance" (1981).

10. H. Ginsburg and S. Opper, *Piaget's Theory of Intellectual Development* (1969), pp. 155–77. See also J.L. Phillips, Jr., "The Origins of Intellect: Piaget's Theory (Introduction)," in Notterman, ed., *Readings*, pp. 171–79.

11. Phillips, in Notterman, *Readings*, pp. 172–73 (emphasis in original).

12. F.J. Mandriota, D.E. Mintz, and J.M. Notterman, "Visual Velocity Discrimination: Effects of Spatial and Temporal Cues" (1962).

13. Ibid. The quasi-random combination is more difficult to judge than either the isochronal or isometric (equal distance). The isochronal is best.

14. J.M. Notterman, R.D.L. Filion, and F.J. Mandriota, "Perception of Changes in Certain Exteroceptive Stimuli" (1971). See also J.M. Notterman and J. Farley, "Experimental Psychology: Recent Developments," in B.B. Wolman, ed., *International Encyclopedia of Psychiatry, Psychology, Psychoanalysis, and Neurology*, Progress vol. 1 (1983).

15. E.A. Alluisi and B.B. Morgan, Jr., "Engineering Psychology and Human Performance," in Rosenzweig and Porter, eds., *Annual Review of Psychology* (1976).

16. E.C. Poulton, *Tracking Skill and Manual Control* (1974).

17. J.M. Notterman and D.O. Weitzman, "Organization and Learning of Visual-Motor Information during Different Orders of Limb Movement" (1981). See also J.M. Notterman, D.R. Tufano, and J.S. Hrapsky, "Visual-Motor Organization: Differences Between and Within Individuals" (1982).

18. D.A. Norman, "Twelve Issues for Cognitive Science" (1980).

19. M.I. Posner, "Coordination of Internal Codes," in W.G. Chase, ed., *Visual Information Processing* (1973).

20. Notterman, Tufano, and Hrapsky, "Visual-Motor Organization" (1982).

21. Battig has made a similar argument concerning the existence of within-individual differences, but in the context of verbal learning. See W.F. Battig, "Within-Indi-

vidual Differences in 'Cognitive' Processes," in R.L. Solso, ed., *Information Processing and Cognition: The Loyola Symposium* (1975).

4. Associationism: Philosophical, Experimental, and Clinical Approaches

    1. G. Murphy and J.K. Kovach, *Historical Introduction to Modern Psychology* (1972), p. 13.

    2. W.A. Rosenblith, "On Cybernetics and the Human Brain," in Notterman, *Readings*, pp. 229–38.

    3. Ibid., p. 231.

    4. J.O. de la Mettrie, *L'Homme Machine* (1748), excerpted in Herrnstein and Boring, *Source Book*, p. 273 (emphasis added).

    5. J. Locke, *An Essay Concerning Humane Understanding* (1700), excerpted in Herrnstein and Boring, p. 338 (emphasis in original).

    6. Ibid., p. 334.

    7. J. Mill, *Analysis of the Phenomena of the Human Mind* (1829) excerpted in Herrnstein and Boring, p. 364.

    8. Ibid., p. 364.

    9. Ibid.

    10. Ibid.

    11. Ibid., p. 365.

    12. Ibid., p. 367 (emphasis added).

    13. D.N. Robinson, *Toward a Science of Human Nature* (1982), p. 19.

    14. J.S. Mill, *A System of Logic* (1843), excerpted in Herrnstein and Boring, p. 380.

    15. D. Schultz, *A History of Modern Psychology* (3d ed., 1981), pp. 73–74.

    16. E.L. Thorndike, "Animal Intelligence: An Experimental Study of the Associative Processes in Animals" (1898), p. 15.

    17. Keller and Schoenfeld, *Principles of Psychology*, p. 39.

    18. Thorndike (1898), cited by D.P. Schultz, *A History of Modern Psychology* (1st ed., 1969), p. 177.

5. Russian Dialectical-Materialist Psychology: Prerevolutionary, Revolutionary, and Postrevolutionary Times

    1. Georg Hegel was a German philosopher (1770–1831), and is considered to be one of the most influential in modern European thought.

    2. The account of dialectical materialism here presented is a consolidation of statements appearing in various reference works (e.g., K.N. Kornilov, "Psychology in the Light of Dialectic Materialism," in C. Murchison, ed., *Psychologies of 1930* [1930], pp. 243–78); articles (e.g., G. Razran, "Soviet Psychology and Psychophysiology" (1958); and dictionaries.

    3. I.M. Sechenov, *Reflexes of the Brain* (1863), excerpted in Herrnstein and Boring, p. 317.

    4. Recall that James Mill, too, was taken with politics.

    5. Sechenov, in Herrnstein and Boring, p. 317. The word "optico" is added, as is the emphasis upon "written."

6. J. Dewey, "The Reflex Arc Concept in Psychology" (1896), excerpted in Herrnstein and Boring, p. 325.

7. Kornilov, Murchison, ed., pp. 263–69 (emphasis in original).

8. G. Razran, "Konstantin Nikolaevich Kornilov, 1879–1957: An Obituary" (1958).

9. A.R. Luria, "Speech Development and the Formation of Mental Processes," in M. Cole and I. Maltzman, eds., A Handbook of Contemporary Soviet Psychology (1969).

10. B.F. Lomov, "Soviet Psychology: Its Historical Origin and Contemporary Status" (1982), p. 582.

11. I.P. Pavlov, quoted in J.F. Fulton, Physiology of the Nervous System (3d ed., 1949), p. 537 (emphasis added).

12. Notterman, Behavior (1970), p. 65.

13. I.P. Pavlov, Lectures on Conditioned Reflexes (1928), excerpted in Herrnstein and Boring, pp. 567–88. The quote is from his speech accepting the Nobel Prize, 1904.

14. H.M. Jenkins and B.R. Moore, "The Form of the Auto-Shaped Response with Food or Water Reinforcers" (1973), p. 179.

15. R.S. Woodworth and M.R. Sheehan, Contemporary Schools of Psychology (3d ed., 1964), p. 79 (emphasis in original).

16. However, trace conditioning appears consistently to produce a heart-rate depression in human subjects. See J.M. Notterman, W.N. Schoenfeld, and P.J. Bersh, "Conditioned Heart Rate Response in Human Subjects during Experimental Anxiety" (1952).

17. Skinner discusses Konorski and Miller's research in The Behavior of Organisms (1938), p. 112. His remarks are of special interest in light of what is now called "biofeedback." See also Keller and Schoenfeld, pp. 62–64.

18. G. Razran, "The Observable Unconscious and the Inferable Conscious in Current Soviet Psychophysiology" (1961), pp. 81–147.

19. N.N. Ladygina-Kots and Y.N. Dembovski, "The Psychology of Primates," in Cole and Maltzman, pp. 53–58.

20. A.V. Zaporozhets, "Origin and Development of Conscious Control of Movements in Man" (1960).

21. Luria, in Cole and Maltzman, pp. 121–28.

22. Notterman, Schoenfeld, and Bersh, "A Comparison of Three Extinction Procedures Following Heart Rate Conditioning" (1952).

23. N.A. Bernshtein, "Methods for Developing Physiology as Related to the Problems of Cybernetics," in Cole and Maltzman, pp. 441–45.

24. Ibid., p. 443.

6. American Behaviorism: Watsonian and Skinnerian Versions

1. J.B. Watson, "Psychology as the Behaviorist Views It" (1913).

2. Schultz (3d ed., 1981), p. 227. The book referred to is Behaviorism (1925).

3. American Psychological Association Monitor (1975), vol. 6, no. 8.

4. Watson, "Psychology as the Behaviorist Views It" (1913), excerpted in Herrnstein and Boring, p. 513 (emphasis in original). The next three quotations appear on pp. 513–14. The fifth quotation is from p. 507.

5. Woodworth and Sheehan, p. 113.

6. Skinner (1938), p. 6 (emphasis added).

7. Skinner, pp. 6–7.

8. Skinner (7th printing, 1966), Preface, p. x.

9. Skinner, p. 4 (emphasis added).

10. Skinner, "The Steep and Thorny Way to a Science of Behavior" (1975), p. 42.

11. J.M. Notterman and D.E. Mintz, *Dynamics of Response* (1965).

12. Notterman and Tufano (1980); Notterman, Tufano, and Hrapsky (1982).

13. Jenkins and Moore (1973), p. 104.

14. Ibid. Wolin's research is briefly described.

15. Ibid., p. 164 (sentences inverted).

16. Notterman and Mintz (1965).

17. D.E. Mintz, "Force of Response during Ratio Reinforcement" (1962).

18. Skinner (1938), p. 338.

19. Notterman and Mintz, "Exteroceptive Cueing of Response Force" (1962).

20. Ibid., p. 1070.

21. Ibid., p. 1071.

22. Notterman and Mintz (1965), pp. 115–18. The investigators show that rate of bar pressing is related by a power function to rate of reinforcement, and that rate of reinforcement—in turn—is a joint function of rate and accuracy of bar pressing.

23. Skinner, *Beyond Freedom and Dignity* (1971).

24. N. Chomsky, Review of B.F. Skinner, *Beyond Freedom and Dignity* (1971).

25. Skinner, "Selection by Consequences" (1981), p. 504.

26. L. Edel, "Portrait of the Artist as an Old Man" (1978), p. 62 (emphasis in original).

7. Gestalt Psychology: Psychophysical Isomorphism and Insight-Thinking

1. W. Kohler, *Gestalt Psychology* (1929), p. 47.

2. C.C. Pratt, Introduction to W. Kohler, *The Task of Gestalt Psychology* (1969), p. 10 (emphasis in original).

3. I.M. Spigel, "Problems in the Study of Visually Perceived Movement: An Introduction," in Spiegel, ed., *Readings in the Study of Visually Perceived Movement* (1965); quotation is from pp. 1–2.

4. Kohler, *The Task of Gestalt Psychology;* p. 66.

5. Ibid., p. 93.

6. Ibid. (punctuation added).

7. D. Brenner, S.J. Williamson, and L. Kauffman, "Visually Evoked Magnetic Fields of the Human Brain" (1975).

8. Kohler, *The Task of Gestalt Psychology,* p. 133 (emphasis added).

9. Ibid., pp. 133–34. Wertheimer's *Productive Thinking* (1945) was published posthumously.

10. Ibid., p. 157.

11. Ladygina-Kots and Dembovskii, in Cole and Maltzman (1969), p. 64.

12. Ibid., p. 41. The quotation appears on p. 63.

13. Notterman, Tufano, and Hrapsky (1982).

14. Ladygina-Kots and Dembovskii, p. 44.

15. H.S. Terrace, L.A. Petitto, R.J. Sanders, and T.G. Bever, "Can an Ape Create a Sentence?" (1979).

16. S. Harnad, ed., "A Special Issue on Cognition and Consciousness in Non-human Species," *Behavioral and Brain Sciences* (1978), vol. 1.
17. W.A. Mason, "Environmental Models and Mental Modes: Representational Processes in the Great Apes and Man" (1976).
18. Woodworth and Sheehan, p. 230.

8. Freudian Psychoanalysis: Major Concepts and Their Relation to Conventional Variables

1. Portions of this chapter are after Notterman, *Behavior* (1970).
2. *The Random House Dictionary of the English Language, Unabridged* (1967).
3. Freud, *New Introductory Lectures on Psychoanalysis* (1932), p. 103, cited by Woodworth and Sheehan, pp. 282–83.
4. C.S. Hall and G. Lindzey, *Theories of Personality* (1957), p. 34.
5. Ibid., p. 34.
6. Ibid., p. 55.
7. From B.B. Wolman, *Dictionary of Behavioral Science* (1973), with slight word changes.
8. D. Bakan, *Sigmund Freud and the Jewish Mystical Tradition* (1958).
9. Ibid., p. 259.
10. J. Nelson, "A Study in Dreams" (1887), p. 375.
11. E.R. Hilgard, *Theories of Learning* (1956), p. 291.
12. R.F. Hefferline, B. Keenan, and R.A. Harford, "Escape and Avoidance Conditioning in Human Subjects Without Their Observation of the Response" (1959).

9. The Challenges to Psychoanalytic Theory and Therapy: Neo-Freudian and Behavioristic Dissent

1. Wolman, *Dictionary*, p. 328.
2. Hall and Lindzey, p. 80.
3. G. Victor, "Interpretations Couched in Mythical Imagery" (1978). Quote is from footnote 1, pp. 237–38.
4. Ibid., p. 231.
5. Woodworth and Sheehan, p. 311.
6. A.K. Adler, "Adler, Alfred (1870–1937)," in Wolman, ed., *International Encyclopedia of Psychiatry, Psychology, Psychoanalysis, and Neurology*, (1977), vol. 1, p. 238.
7. Wolman, *Dictionary*, p. 115.
8. Ibid., p. 220.
9. Ibid., p. 191.
10. After Woodworth and Sheehan, p. 329.
11. See Woodworth and Sheehan, pp. 330–31, for an excellent brief description of Sullivan's "modes." The studies of Solomon Asch ("Opinions and Social Pressure," *Scientific American*, November 1955) are considered classics in the field of conformity. They are summarized in Notterman, *Behavior* (1970), pp. 319–24.
12. R.R. Grinker, "A Philosophical Appraisal of Psychoanalysis," in J.H. Masserman, ed., *Science and Psychoanalysis* (1958), vol. 1, p. 132.
13. H.L. Silverman, "Jung: Historical and Methodological Considerations," in

Wolman, ed., *International Encyclopedia of Psychiatry, Psychology, Psychoanalysis, and Neurology* (1977), vol. 6, p. 230.

14. Keller and Schoenfeld, *Principles of Psychology* (1950), p. 138.

15. Ibid., p. 310.

16. J. Wolpe refined these propositions in his seminal book, *Psychotherapy by Reciprocal Inhibition* (1958).

17. R. Moore, "Imprisoning Abstractions" (1974).

18. G.T. Wilson and A.A. Lazarus, "Behavior Modification and Therapy," in Wolman, ed., *The Therapist's Handbook* (2d ed., 1983), p. 140.

19. J. Marmor and S.M. Woods, eds., *The Interface between the Psychodynamic and Behavioral Therapies* (1980). See also Wolman's *The Therapist's Handbook*.

10. Epilogue and Prologue: Four Enduring Issues, and the Future of Psychology

1. S. Arieti, "Presidential Address: Psychoanalytic Therapy in a Cultural Climate of Pessimism" (1981).

Bibliography

Adler, A.K. "Adler, Alfred (1870–1937)." In B.B. Wolman, ed., *International Encyclopedia of Psychiatry, Psychology, Psychoanalysis, and Neurology*, vol. 1. New York: Van Nostrand Reinhold, 1977.

Alluisi, E.A. and B.B. Morgan, Jr. "Engineering Psychology and Human Performance." In M.R. Rosenzweig and L.W. Porter, eds., *Annual Review of Psychology*. Palo Alto, Cal.: Annual Reviews, 1976.

Arieti, S. "Presidential Address: Psychoanalytic Therapy in a Climate of Pessimism." *Journal of the American Academy of Psychoanalysis* (1981), 9:171–84.

Bakan, D. *Sigmund Freud and the Jewish Mystical Tradition*. Princeton: Van Nostrand, 1958.

Battig, W.F. "Within-Individual Differences in 'Cognitive' Processes." In R.L. Solso, ed., *Information Processing and Cognition: The Loyola Symposium*. Hillsdale, N.J.: Erlbaum, 1975.

Bernshtein, N.A. "Methods for Developing Physiology as Related to the Problems of Cybernetics." In M. Cole and I. Maltzman, eds., *A Handbook of Contemporary Soviet Psychology*. New York: Basic Books, 1969.

Brenner, D., S.J. Williamson, and L. Kauffman. "Visually Evoked Magnetic Fields of the Human Brain." *Science* (1975), 187:480–82.

Brett, G.S. *A History of Psychology: Ancient and Patristic*, vol. 1. London: George Allen & Unwin, 1912.

Carrington, R. *A Guide to Earth History*. New York: Harper, 1956.

Chomsky, N. Review of B.F. Skinner, *Beyond Freedom and Dignity*. *The New York Review of Books* (1971), 17:18–24.

Dewey, J. "The Reflex Arc Concept in Psychology" (excerpt). In R.J. Herrstein and E.G. Boring, eds., *A Source Book in the History of Psychology*. Cambridge, Mass.: Harvard University Press, 1968.

Durant, W. *The Story of Philosophy*. New York: Simon & Schuster, 1926.

Edel, L. "Portrait of the Artist as an Old Man." *American Scholar* (Winter 1977/78), 47:52–68.

Freud, S. *Totem and Taboo*. In A.A. Brill, ed., *Basic Writings of Sigmund Freud*. New York: Basic Books, 1938.

——*Moses and Monotheism.* In J. Strachey, ed., *The Complete Psychological Works of Sigmund Freud,* vol. 23. London: The Hogarth Press, 1964.

Fulton, J.F. *Physiology of the Nervous System,* 3d ed. New York: Oxford University Press, 1949.

Ginsburg, H. and S. Opper. *Piaget's Theory of Intellectual Development.* Englewood Cliffs, N.J.: Prentice-Hall, 1969.

Grinker, R.R. "A Philosophical Appraisal of Psychoanalysis." In J.H. Masserman, ed., *Science and Psychoanalysis,* vol. 1. New York: Grune & Stratton, 1958.

Hall, C.S. and G. Lindzey. *Theories of Personality.* New York: Wiley, 1957.

Harnad, S., ed. "A Special Issue on Cognition and Consciousness in Nonhuman Species." *Behavioral and Brain Sciences* (1978), 1:515–629.

Hartzell, D.J. *Odysseus: The Complete Adventures.* Wellesley Hills, Mass. The Independent School Press, 1978.

Hefferline, R.F., B. Keenan, and R.A. Harford. "Escape and Avoidance Conditioning in Human Subjects Without Their Observation of the Response." *Science* (1959), 130:1338–39.

Heidbreder, E. *Seven Psychologies.* New York: Appleton-Century, 1932.

Hilgard, E.R. *Theories of Learning.* New York: Appleton-Century-Crofts, 1956.

—— "Consciousness in Contemporary Psychology." In M.R. Rosenzweig and L.W. Porter, eds., *Annual Review of Psychology.* Palo Alto, Cal.: Annual Reviews, 1980.

Homer. *The Complete Works of Homer.* New York: Random House (The Modern Library), 1950.

Hrapsky, J.S. "Effects of Training in Visual Observation upon Subsequent Visual-Motor Performance." Ph.D. diss., Princeton University, 1981.

James, W. *The Principles of Psychology* (excerpt). In R.J. Herrnstein and E.G. Boring, eds., *A Source Book in the History of Psychology.* Cambridge, Mass.: Harvard University Press, 1968.

Jaynes, J.J. *The Origin of Consciousness in the Breakdown of the Bicameral Mind.* Boston: Houghton Mifflin, 1977.

Jenkins, H.M. and B.R. Moore, "The Form of the Auto-Shaped Response with Food or Water Reinforcers." *Journal of the Experimental Analysis of Behavior* (1973), 20:163–81.

Keller, F.S. and W.N. Schoenfeld. *Principles of Psychology.* New York: Appleton-Century-Crofts, 1950.

Kohler, W. *Gestalt Psychology.* New York: Liveright, 1929.

—— *The Task of Gestalt Psychology.* Princeton, N.J.: Princeton University Press, 1969.

Kornilov, K.N. "Psychology in the Light of Dialectic Materialism." In C. Murchison, ed., *Psychologies of 1930.* Worcester, Mass.: Clark University Press, 1930.

Ladygina-Kots, N.N. and Y.N. Dembovskii. "The Psychology of Primates." In M. Cole and I. Maltzman, eds., *A Handbook of Contemporary Soviet Psychology.* New York: Basic Books, 1969.

La Mettrie, J.O. de. *L'Homme Machine* (excerpt). In R.J. Herrnstein and E.G. Boring, eds., *A Source Book in the History of Psychology.* Cambridge, Mass.: Harvard University Press, 1968.

Langfeld, H.S. "A Response Interpretation of Consciousness." *Psychological Review* (1931), 38:87–95.

Locke, J. *An Essay Concerning Humane Understanding* (excerpt). In R.J. Herrnstein and E.G. Boring, eds., *A Source Book in the History of Psychology*. Cambridge, Mass.: Harvard University Press, 1968.

Lomov, B.F. "Soviet Psychology: Its Historical Origins and Contemporary Status." *American Psychologist* (1982), 37:580–86.

Luria, A.R. "Speech Development and the Formation of Mental Processes." In M. Cole and I. Maltzman, eds., *A Handbook of Contemporary Soviet Psychology*. New York: Basic Books, 1969.

Mandriota, F.J., D.E. Mintz, and J.M. Notterman. "Visual Velocity Discrimination: Effects of Spatial and Temporal Cues." *Science* (1962), 138:437–38.

Marmor, J. and S.M. Woods, eds. *The Interface between the Psychodynamic and Behavioral Therapies*. New York: Plenum, 1980.

Marshack, A. *Ice Age Art: 35,000–10,000 B.C.* New York: American Museum of Natural History, 1978.

Maslow, A.H. "A Philosophy of Psychology: The Need for a Mature Science of Human Nature." In F.T. Severin, ed., *Humanistic Viewpoints in Psychology*. New York: McGraw-Hill, 1965.

Mason, W.A. "Environmental Models and Mental Modes: Representational Processes in the Great Apes and Man." *American Psychologist* (1976), 31:284–94.

McDougall, W. *Outline of Psychology* (excerpt). In R.J. Herrnstein and E.G. Boring, eds., *A Source Book in the History of Psychology*. Cambridge, Mass.: Harvard University Press, 1968.

Mill, J. *Analysis of the Phenomena of the Human Mind* (excerpt). In R.J. Herrnstein and E.G. Boring, eds., *A Source Book in the History of Psychology*. Cambridge, Mass.: Harvard University Press, 1968.

Mill, J.S. *A System of Logic* (excerpt). In R.J. Herrnstein and E.G. Boring, eds., *A Source Book in the History of Psychology*. Cambridge, Mass.: Harvard University Press, 1968.

Miller, G.A. *Mathematics and Psychology*. New York: Wiley, 1964.

Mintz, D.E. "Force of Response during Ratio Reinforcement." *Science* (1962), 138:516–17.

Moore, R. "Imprisoning Abstractions." *Contemporary Psychoanalysis* (1974), 10:503–10.

Murphy, G. *Historical Introduction to Modern Psychology*. New York: Harcourt, Brace, 1949.

Murphy, G. and J.K. Kovach. *Historical Introduction to Modern Psychology*. New York: Harcourt Brace Jovanovich, 1972.

Nagel, E. "Self Regulation." In D. Flanagan, ed., *Automatic Control*. New York: Simon and Schuster, 1955.

Nelson, J. "A Study in Dreams." *American Journal of Psychology* (1887), 1:367–401.

Norman, D.A. "Twelve Issues for Cognitive Science." *Cognitive Science* (1980), 4:1–32.

Notterman, J.M. *Behavior: A Systematic Approach.* New York: Random House, 1970.

—— "Discussion of On-line Computers in the Animal Laboratory." *Behavioral Research Methods and Instrumentation* (1973), 5:129–31.

Notterman, J.M. and J. Farley. "Experimental Psychology: Recent Developments." In B.B. Wolman, ed., *International Encyclopedia of Psychiatry, Psychology, Psychoanalysis, and Neurology.* Progress vol. 1. New York: Aesculapius, 1983.

Notterman, J.M., R.D.L. Filion, and F.J. Mandriota. "Perception of Changes in Certain Exteroceptive Stimuli." *Science* (1971), 173:1206–11.

Notterman, J.M. and D.E. Mintz. "Exteroceptive Cueing of Response Force." *Science* (1962), 135:1070–71.

—— *Dynamics of Response.* New York: Wiley, 1965.

Notterman, J.M., W.N. Schoenfeld, and P.J. Bersh. "A Comparison of Three Extinction Procedures Following Heart Rate Conditioning." *Journal of Abnormal and Social Psychology* (1952), 47:674–77.

—— "Conditioned Heart Rate Response in Human Subjects during Experimental Anxiety." *Journal of Comparative and Physiological Psychology* (1952), 45:1–8.

Notterman, J.M. and D.R. Tufano. "Variables Influencing Outflow-Inflow Interpretations of Tracking Performance: Predictability of Target Motion, Transfer Function, and Practice." *Journal of Experimental Psychology: Human Perception and Performance* (1980), 6:85–88.

Notterman, J.M., D.R. Tufano, and J.S. Hrapsky. "Visual-Motor Organization: Differences Between and Within Individuals." *Perceptual and Motor Skills* (1982), 54:723–50 (Monograph Supplement 2-V54).

Notterman, J.M. and D.O. Weitzman. "Organization and Learning of Visual-Motor Information during Different Orders of Limb Movement: Step, Velocity, Acceleration." *Journal of Experimental Psychology: Human Perception and Performance* (1981), 7:916–27.

Pavlov, I.P. *Lectures on Conditioned Reflexes* (excerpt). In R.J. Herrnstein and E.G. Boring, eds., *A Source in the History of Psychology.* Cambridge, Mass.: Harvard University Press, 1968.

Pfeiffer, J.E. *The Emergence of Man.* New York: Harper & Row, 1972.

Phillips, J.L., Jr. *The Origins of Intellectual Development: Piaget's Theory* (Introduction). In J.M. Notterman, ed. *Readings in Behavior.* New York: Random House, 1970.

Posner, M.I. "Coordination of Internal Codes." In W.G. Chase, ed., *Visual Information Processing.* New York: Academic Press, 1973.

Poulton, E.C. *Tracking Skill and Manual Control.* New York: Academic Press, 1974.

Random House Dictionary of the English Language, Unabridged. New York: Random House, 1967.

Razran, G. "Konstantin Nikolaevich Kornilov, 1879–1957: An Obituary." *Science* (1958), 128:74–75.

—— "Soviet Psychology and Psychophysiology." *Science* (1958), 128: 1187–94.

—— "The Observable Unconscious and the Inferable Conscious in Current Soviet Psychophysiology." *Psychological Review* (1961), 68:81–147.

Robinson, D.N. *The Enlightened Machine.* New York: Columbia University Press, 1980.

—— *Toward a Science of Human Nature.* New York: Columbia University Press, 1982.

Rosenblith, W.A. "On Cybernetics and the Human Brain." In J.M. Notterman, ed., *Readings in Behavior.* New York: Random House, 1970.

Rosenblueth, A., N. Weiner, and J. Bigelow. "Behavior, Purpose, and Teleology." In J.M. Notterman, ed., *Readings in Behavior.* New York: Random House, 1970.

Schultz, D. *A History of Modern Psychology,* 3d edition. New York: Academic Press, 1981.

Sechenov, I.M. *Reflexes of the Brain* (excerpt). In R.J. Herrnstein and E.G. Boring, eds., *A Source Book in the History of Psychology.* Cambridge, Mass.: Harvard University Press, 1968.

Silverman, H.L. "Jung: Historical and Methodological Considerations." In B.B. Wolman, ed., *International Encyclopedia of Psychiatry, Psychology, Psychoanalysis, and Neurology,* vol. 6. New York: Van Nostrand Rheinhold, 1977.

Skinner, B.F. *The Behavior of Organisms: An Experimental Analysis.* New York: Appleton-Century, 1938.

—— *Beyond Freedom and Dignity.* New York: Knopf, 1971.

—— "The Steep and Thorny Way to a Science of Behavior." *American Psychologist* (1975), 30:42–49.

—— "Selection by Consequences." *Science* (1981), 213:501–4.

Spiegel, I.M. "Problems in the Study of Visually Perceived Movement: An Introduction." In I.M. Spigel, ed., *Readings in the Study of Visually Perceived Movement.* New York: Harper & Row, 1965.

Tart, C.T. "States of Consciousness and State-Specific Sciences." *Science* (1972), 176:1203–10.

Terrace, H.S., L.A. Petitto, R.J. Sanders, and T.G. Bever. "Can an Ape Create a Sentence?" *Science* (1979), 206:891–92.

Thorndike, E.L. "Animal Intelligence: An Experimental Study of the Associative Processes in Animals." *Psychological Review Supplements* (1898), 2(4), whole no. 8.

Titchener, E.B. *An Outline of Psychology.* New York: Macmillan, 1896.

Victor, G. "Interpretations Couched in Mythical Imagery." *Journal of Psychoanalytic Psychotherapy* (1978), 7:225–39.

Watson, J.B. "Psychology as the Behaviorist Views It." *Psychological Review* (1913), 20:158–77.

—— "Psychology as the Behaviorist Views It" (excerpt). In R.J. Herrnstein and E.G. Boring, eds., *A Source Book in the History of Psychology.* Cambridge, Mass.: Harvard University Press, 1968.

Wiener, N. *Cybernetics.* New York: Wiley, 1948.

Wilson, G.T. and A.A. Lazarus. "Behavior Modification and Therapy." In B.B. Wolman, ed., *The Therapist's Handbook: Treatment Methods of Mental Disorders,* 2d ed. New York: Van Nostrand Reinhold, 1983.

Wolman, B.B. *Dictionary of Behavioral Science.* New York: Van Nostrand Reinhold, 1973.

Wolman, B.B., ed. *The Therapist's Handbook: Treatment Methods of Mental Disorders*, 2d ed. New York: Van Nostrand Reinhold, 1983.

Wolpe, J. *Psychotherapy by Reciprocal Inhibition*. Stanford, Cal.: Stanford University Press, 1958.

Woodworth, R.S. "Dynamic Psychology." In C. Murchison, ed., *Psychologies of 1930*. Worcester, Mass.: Clark University Press, 1930.

—— *Experimental Psychology*. New York: Holt, 1938.

—— and M.R. Sheehan. *Contemporary Schools of Psychology*. 3d ed. New York: Ronald Press, 1964.

World Almanac & Book of Facts. New York: Newspaper Enterprise Association, 1984.

Zaporozhets, A.V. "Origin and Development of Conscious Control of Movements in Man." In *The Central Nervous System and Behavior: Translations from the Russian Medical Literature*. Bethesda, Md.: National Institutes of Health, U.S. Public Health Service, 1960.

Index

Critical Assessments of Contemporary Psychology
Daniel N. Robinson, Series Editor